Neonatal Pain
Suffering, Pain and Risk of Brain Damage in the Fetus and Newborn

GU00982591

Giuseppe Buonocore • Carlo V. Bellieni

Editors

Neonatal Pain
Suffering, Pain and Risk of Brain Damage in the Fetus and Newborn

Foreword by Ignacio Carrasco de Paula

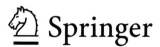 Springer

Giuseppe Buonocore
Department of Pediatrics, Obstetrics and
Reproduction Medicine
University of Siena
Siena, Italy

Carlo V. Bellieni
Department of Pediatrics, Obstetrics and
Reproduction Medicine
University of Siena
Siena, Italy

Cover illustration: Leonardo da Vinci, The Babe in the Womb, c. 1511 (detail).
The Royal Collection © 2007 Her Majesty Queen Elizabeth II

Library of Congress Control Number: 2007938688

ISBN 978-88-470-0731-4 Springer Milan Berlin Heidelberg New York
e-ISBN 978-88-470-0732-1

Springer is a part of Springer Science+Business Media

© Springer-Verlag Italia 2008

springer.com

Cover design: Simona Colombo, Milan, Italy
Typesetting: C & G di Cerri e Galassi, Cremona, Italy
Printing: Arti Grafiche Nidasio, Assago (MI), Italy

Printed in Italy
Springer-Verlag Italia S.r.l. – Via Decembrio 28 – I-20137 Milan

Preface

For many years we have been talking about a very special patient, the embryo; and the numerous and encouraging successes brought about by embryofetal medicine in the application of both noninvasive therapies and invasive ultrasound-guided treatment are well known.

On the other hand, it is more and more often the case today that the small patients in neonatal care are premature babies who have come to the world at a particularly low gestational age. This allows us to observe the continuity between the phases of growth inside the maternal uterus and after birth, which arrives at the correct moment for some lucky fetuses, for others very early, and for some altogether too soon. The neonatologists have the arduous task of sustaining these little patients in their strivings to survive, registering their energy and their vital dynamism, studying the progressive development of the anatomical structures and the improvement of their physiology, verifying day by day the presence – sometimes fragile, sometimes extremely resistant, but always human – of a child.

A long line research has shown how, from the first moment onwards in that process of perfectly coordinated development that characterizes the life of the embryo, a human being gradually emerges who is increasingly able to interact with his or her environment. Despite neurosensory immaturity, some unsuspected perceptive abilities have been found in the fetus, particularly in regard to the perception of pain, which can be also deeper in the following phases of development, that is, in the child once it has been born. However, the large amount of scientific evidence attesting to the fact that the fetus can already feel pain around halfway through the pregnancy have not been welcomed by the international scientific community; in fact, very varying positions are recorded, with inevitable consequences at both the clinical and the ethical level.

The issue of fetal pain is one of the so-called border subjects, which go well over the positive data of the experimental study to involve the minds and consciences of those contemplating it, arousing opposing reactions and discordant opinions. In the political arena too, the issue of fetal pain has been enlisted on one side or the other or given rise to controversies, as has been recently seen in USA. If the scientific data are accompanied with resistance and interpretation, it is evident, in some cases, that people will select their data depending on which way they want to argue, in favour of a particular thesis.

The controversies that have arisen in some states in the USA are due to the decision to anaesthetize the fetus before a voluntary interruption of pregnancy, while reading to the mother a document explaining that the fetus feels pain. Some political exponents have interpreted this as an initiative to discourage women who have decided to abort. But we cannot ignore scientific work, including that published by the authors of this volume, showing that the fetus is able to perceive pain because it is already in possession of sufficiently developed anatomical structures, and that it is able to give some physiological and behavioural responses after painful stimuli. The difference between "nociception", verifiable by accurate studies, and "conscious recognition of a painful stimulus" is therefore of primary importance: it is on this last element that some positions rely when denying, in a not very deep way, how much is indeed verifiable in the investigations published in the present book. Talking about the consciousness of pain may be a bit nebulous when it is done in regard to contexts where it is hardly verifiable. The perception of painful stimuli and their relative transmission to the superior nervous centres, on the other hand, is well documented. Furthermore, the influence on the future life of the child of extended painful stimuli received in the fetal and neonatal stage has been demonstrated. It is in this wide-ranging way, with the future child kept always in view, that the scientific studies must be appraised: taking this approach, the opportunity to consider analgesia in the fetus is obvious.

The studies described in this book tend in this direction, allowing us to get to know the fetus better as a patient, and dealing with the delicate matter of its treatment. Fetal analgesia is an area full of future developments that are not without ethical implications. What seems to be fundamental in this field is to confirm that the exclusive interest of the patient and respect for human dignity must always be kept at the forefront in studies in humans and the application of their results.

Rome, December 2007   *Ignacio Carrasco de Paula, MD PhD*
                                                     Department of Bioethics
                                                     Faculty of Medicine and Surgery
                                                     A. Gemelli Hospital
                                                     Catholic University of the Sacred Heart
                                                     Rome

Contents

List of Contributors

Anna M. Aloisi
Pain and Stress Neurophysiology Lab, Department of Physiology, University of Siena, Siena, Italy

Aldo Altomare
Section of Obstetrics and Gynecology, Department of Pediatrics, Obstetrics and Reproductive Medicine, University of Siena, Siena, Italy

Giovanna Amato
Section of Pediatric Surgery, Department of Pediatrics, Obstertrics and Reproductive Medicine, University of Siena, Siena, Italy

Kanwaljeet S. Anand
Department of Pediatrics, University of Arkansas for Medical Sciences, Arkansas Children's Hospital, Little Rock, Arkansas, USA

Paolo Arosio
Neonatology, Neonatal Intensive Therapy Unit, San Gerardo Hospital, Monza, Italy

Emanuele Basile
Department of Child Psychiatry Eugenio Medea, Scientific Institute, Bosisio Parini, Lecco, Italy

Raffaele Battista
Division of Obstetrics and Gynecology, Department of Pediatrics, Obstetrics and Reproductive Medicine, University of Siena, Siena, Italy

Carlo V. Bellieni
Department of Pediatrics, Obstetrics and Reproduction Medicine, University of Siena, Siena, Italy

Chiara Benedetto
Chair C of the Department of Obstetrics and Gynaecology, University of Turin, Turin, Italy

Silvia Blefari
Chair C of the Department of Obstetrics and Gynaecology, University of Turin, Turin, Italy

Caterina Bocchi
Section of Obstetrics and Gynecology, Department of Pediatrics, Obstetrics and Reproductive Medicine, University of Siena, Siena, Italy

Carlotta Boni
Section of Obstetrics and Gynecology, Department of Pediatrics, Obstetrics and Reproductive Medicine, University of Siena, Siena, Italy

Luca Bonino
Chair C of the Department of Obstetrics and Gynaecology, University of Turin, Turin, Italy

Luca Bruni
Section of Obstetrics and Gynecology, Department of Pediatrics, Obstetrics and Reproductive Medicine, University of Siena, Siena, Italy

Giuseppe Buonocore
Department of Pediatrics, Obstetrics and Reproduction Medicine, University of Siena, Siena, Italy

Ricardo Carbajal
Centre National de Ressources de Lutte contre la Douleur, Hôpital d'Enfants Armand Trousseau, Paris, France

Alessandro Caruso
Department of Obstetrics and Gynecology, Catholic University of Sacred Heart, Rome, Italy

Ilaria Ceccarelli
Pain and Stress Neurophysiology Lab, Department of Physiology, University of Siena, Siena, Italy

Elena Cesari
Department of Obstetrics and Gynecology, Catholic University of Sacred Heart, Rome, Italy

Maria De Bonis
Division of Obstetrics and Gynecology, Department of Pediatrics, Obstetrics and Reproductive Medicine, University of Siena, Siena, Italy

Ada Delia
Section of Obstetrics and Gynecology, Department of Pediatrics, Obstetrics and Reproductive Medicine, University of Siena, Siena, Italy

Maria Delivoria-Papadopoulos
Neonatal Research Laboratory Drexel University College of Medicine, St. Christopher's Hospital for Children, Philadelphia, USA

Arianna Dell'Anna
Division of Obstetrics and Gynecology, Department of Pediatrics, Obstetrics and Reproductive Medicine, University of Siena, Siena, Italy

Catherine Dolto
Department of Pediatrics, Obstetrics and Reproduction Medicine, University of Siena, Italy

Marina Enrichi
Obstetric Psychoprophilaxis Service, Department of Gynecology and Human Reproductive Science, University of Padua, Padua, Italy

Alessandra Ferrarini
Department of Pediatrics, Fondazione Ospedale Maggiore, Mangiagalli e Regina Elena, Milan, Italy
Department of Pediatrics, San Giovanni Hospital, Bellinzona, Switzerland

Caterina Ferretti
Division of Obstetrics and Gynecology, Department of Pediatrics, Obstetrics and Reproductive Medicine, University of Siena, Siena, Italy

Gilda Filardi
Section of Obstetrics and Gynecology, Department of Pediatrics, Obstetrics and Reproductive Medicine, University of Siena, Siena, Italy

Pasquale Florio
Division of Obstetrics and Gynecology, Department of Pediatrics, Obstetrics and Reproductive Medicine, University of Siena, Siena, Italy

Giuseppe P. Fortunato
Department of Obstetrics and Gynecology, Catholic University of Sacred Heart, Rome, Italy

Laura Giuntini
Department of Intensive Care, Policlinic Le Scotte, Siena, Siena, Italy

Vivette Glover
Institute of Reproductive and Developmental Biology, Imperial College London, London, United Kingdom

Evelina Gollo
Department of Anaesthesia, OIRM S. Anna, Turin, Italy

Chiara Greco
Department of Obstetrics and Gynecology, Catholic University of Sacred Heart, Rome, Italy

Anna M. Guadagni
Department of Medical and Surgical Neonatology, Bambin Gesù Pediatric Hospital – I.R.C.C.S. – Roma, Italy

Maria Serena Ligato
Department of Obstetrics and Gynecology, Catholic University of Sacred Heart, Rome, Italy

Stefano Luisi
Division of Obstetrics and Gynecology, Department of Pediatrics, Obstetrics and Reproductive Medicine, University of Siena, Siena, Italy

Ilenia Mappa
Department of Obstetrics and Gynecology, Catholic University of Sacred Heart, Rome, Italy

Luigi Memo
Neonatal Intensive Care Unit, S. Maria di Cà Foncello Hospital, Treviso, Italy

Om P. Mishra
Neonatal Research Laboratory, Drexel University College of Medicine, St. Christopher's Hospital for Children, Philadelphia, USA

Giuseppe Noia
Department of Obstetrics and Gynecology, Catholic University of Sacred Heart, Rome, Italy

Kieran O'Donnell
Institute of Reproductive and Developmental Biology, Imperial College London, London, United Kingdom

Marco Palumbo
Department of Microbiological and Gynecological Science, University of Catania, Siena and Catania, Italy

Felice Petraglia
Division of Obstetrics and Gynecology, Department of Pediatrics, Obstetrics and
Reproductive Medicine, University of Siena, Siena, Italy

Mariachiara Quadrifoglio
Division of Obstetrics and Gynecology, Department of Pediatrics, Obstetrics and
Reproductive Medicine, University of Siena, Siena, Italy

Fernando M. Reis
Division of Obstetrics and Gynecology, Department of Pediatrics, Obstetrics and
Reproductive Medicine, University of Siena, Siena, Italy

Onofrio S. Saia
Neonatal Intensive Care Unit, S. Maria di Cà Foncello Hospital, Treviso, Italy

Angelo Selicorni
Department of Pediatrics, Fondazione Ospedale Maggiore, Mangiagalli e Regina
Elena, Milan, Italy

Filiberto M. Severi
Section of Obstetrics and Gynecology, Department of Pediatrics, Obstetrics and
Reproductive Medicine, University of Siena, Siena, Italy

Renata Sisto
ISPESL, Department of Occupational Hygiene, Monte Porzio Catone, Rome, Italy

Mauro Tintoni
Department of Obstetrics and Gynecology, Catholic University of Sacred Heart,
Rome, Italy

Daniela Visconti
Department of Obstetrics and Gynecology, Catholic University of Sacred Heart,
Rome, Italy

Charles J. Woodbury
Department of Zoology and Physiology, University of Wyoming, Laramie,
Wyoming, USA

Irene Zerbetto
Division of Obstetrics and Gynecology, Department of Pediatrics, Obstetrics and
Reproductive Medicine, University of Siena, Siena, Italy

Marina Zonca
Chair C of the Department of Obstetrics and Gynaecology, University of Turin,
Turin, Italy

Introduction: Pain and Suffering from the Womb Onwards?

G. Buonocore and C.V. Bellieni

What is pain? To paraphrase Augustine of Hippo: "If nobody asks me, I know; if I try to explain it, I don't know" (Confessions 11.14.17).

Pain is the only sensation that we cannot remember. We can remember the stimulus that provoked pain, or its organic consequences, but we cannot recall pain as we recall flavours, noises, and images. It is difficult to describe pain, but we can describe its features, which are of three types:

– The stimulus. We recognize a stimulus as potentially painful even if we cannot see the sufferer's reaction, because we appreciate its intensity and nature (e.g. a lancet on the skin).
– Bodily consequences. Examples are lesions, hormone production (cortisol, endorphins, epinephrine), changes in physiological parameters (heart rate, blood pressure, sweating).
– Behavioural changes.

All three of these features are evident in the case of newborns. Newborns are "psychobiologically social beings" [1] and can feel anxiety and fear. This book will show that they can feel pain even before birth.

But what is "pain" – a term often confused with "suffering"? Cassell wrote: "A search in the medical and social-science literature did not help me in understanding what suffering is: the word 'suffering' was often coupled with the word 'pain', as in 'pain and suffering'" [2]. Although pain and suffering are closely identified in the medical literature, they are phenomenologically distinct. "Pain has a felt quality, a felt intensity. Suffering, on the other hand, is not located in the body" [3], or, "Pain refers to extreme physical distress and comes in many varieties: throbbing, piercing, burning. Suffering, by contrast, refers to a state of psychological burden or oppression, typically marked by fear, dread or anxiety" [4].

"Suffering can be defined as the state of severe distress associated with events that threaten the intactness of the person" [2]. Schopenhauer usefully defined suffering as "the gap between what we demand or expect from life and what actually comes to us" [5] – an idea recently echoed by van Hoof: "Suffering is to be understood as frustration of the tendency towards fulfilment of the various aspects of our being" [6]. Do newborns have desires? Clinical observation of newborns is enough to suggest a nature marked by deep desires: growing, feeding, seeking milk and crying to obtain it are signs of a desire for health [7, 8]. But desires are a person's main

G. Buonocore, C.V. Bellieni (eds), *Neonatal Pain. Suffering, Pain and Risk of Brain Damage in the Fetus and Newborn*, © Springer 2008

1

feature ... are newborns and fetuses persons? Boethius, in his *Liber de persona et duabus naturis*, defined personhood as "an individual substance of rational nature" (*naturae rationalis individua substantia*; Chap. 111, PL 64, 1343), and newborns/fetuses are individuals and with a rational nature, though they do not yet exercise it. Thus it is reasonable to say that newborns and even fetuses are persons, with all their unexpressed desires, and, consequently, suffering.

This book can help us to define what pain and suffering are. Pain is a fundamentally "physical" phenomenon, *the clash arising from an attack on one's physical integrity*, whereas suffering is something broader, with pain as one of its sources and desire as its condition. We can define it as *the clash arising from an attack on the integrity of one's self as a person.*

In conclusion, we can say that newborns and fetuses can feel pain and suffer [9]. This book will show that their personhood becomes more and more evident with the acquisition of progressive skills beginning in prenatal life. Recognizing human dignity and human suffering from life in the womb onwards is a clinical duty in the service of better treatment. This book has been written to overcome anything that would come between an awareness of this fact and the shared effort to provide effective treatment of pain and stress in the preverbal patient.

References

1. Als H, Duffy FH, McAnulty GB (1996) Effectiveness of individualised neurodevelopmental care in the newborn intensive care unit. Acta Paediatr Suppl 416:21–30
2. Cassell EJ (1982) The nature of suffering and the goals of medicine. N Engl J Med 306:639–645
3. Portmann J (1999) Abortion: three rival versions of suffering. Camb Q Healthc Ethics 8:489–497
4. Callahan D (1996) The goals of medicine: setting new priorities. The Hastings Center Report Special Suppl 6:S9–S13
5. Schopenhauer A (1965) On the basis of morality. Trans. Payne EFJ. Indianapolis: Bobbs-Merrill, p 19
6. Van Hoof S (1998) Suffering and the goals of medicine. Med Health Care Philos 1:125–131
7. Bellieni CV, Bagnoli F, Buonocore G (2003) Alone no more: pain in premature children. Ethics Med 19:5–9
8. Bellieni CV, Bagnoli F, Perrone S, et al (2002) Effect of multisensory stimulation on analgesia in term neonates: a randomized controlled trial. Pediatr Res 51:460–463
9. Bellieni C (2005) Pain definitions revised: newborns not only feel pain, they also suffer. Ethics Med 21:5–9

PART I
Delivery and Pain

Chapter 1
Gonadal Hormones and Pain Modulation

A.M. Aloisi and I. Ceccarelli

In a number of animal and human studies, males and females have been shown to differ in their responsiveness to noxious stimuli [1–5]. In humans, many chronic painful syndromes are more common in women than in men. For instance, certain chronic inflammatory conditions, such as rheumatoid arthritis, complex regional pain syndrome and fibromyalgia, have a lower incidence in men than in women [6–9]. Additionally, male rodents typically have higher pain thresholds than females, and gonadectomy lowers the pain threshold in males. There is also a sex difference in the efficacy of the opioids widely used in experimental and clinical studies to test analgesia. For example, male rodents (but not humans) are more sensitive than females to the antinociceptive actions of morphine [10–13].

There could be several reasons for the higher reactivity of females than males to a similar painful stimulus, from genes to hormonal and cultural influences. It is probable that gonadal hormones contribute to these sex differences, because hormone manipulations alter basal nociceptive and analgesic responses. Thus, in our laboratory we concentrate on gonadal hormones, whose receptors are present in many brain areas including some involved in pain transmission and modulation.

Gonadal Hormones, Development and Analgesia

A particular aspect considered in several studies is the development of differences in pain and analgesia mechanisms. The analgesia produced by the stress of swimming in cold water does not differ in magnitude between male and female mice but differs in the underlying mechanisms [14, 15]. Cold water swimming in male mice produces analgesia that can be reversed by the N-methyl-D-aspartate (NMDA) antagonist MK-801, but this is not the case in females. Neonatal exposure of female mice to testosterone results in NMDA-mediated stress-induced analgesia similar to that in males [15].

In another series of studies, Cicero et al. [16] examined how gonadectomy performed neonatally as opposed to in adulthood changes morphine-induced anti-nociception in male rats. Neonatal gonadectomy results in a rightward shift of the morphine dose–response curve compared with that in intact males in the hot plate test.

G. Buonocore, C.V. Bellieni (eds), *Neonatal Pain. Suffering, Pain and Risk of Brain Damage in the Fetus and Newborn*, © Springer 2008

In contrast, the analgesic effect of morphine does not change if gonadectomy is performed in adulthood.

These studies demonstrate that the hormonal milieu early in development helps define the endogenous antinociceptive processes. The neonatal testosterone surge allows masculinization and defeminization of the central nervous system (CNS), including the sex-specific development and distribution of androgen receptors [17, 18]. Testosterone facilitates dendritic growth and neuronal survival [19, 20]. The development of nociceptive pathways may partially depend on the organization and distribution of oestrogen and androgen receptors [21].

In a model of neuropathic pain, LaCroix-Fralish et al. [22] examined both organizational and activational effects of gonadal hormones in male and female rats exposed to painful stimuli. They found that adult circulating hormone levels are critical for the increased sensitivity to mechanical and heat stimulation in females, whereas neonatal or adult gonadectomy does not alter the sensitivity of males.

Borzan and Fuchs [23] investigated the role of testosterone in inflammatory pain by means of intra-articular injections of carrageenan, an animal model of arthritis. They demonstrated that in males the presence of testosterone early in development has an antinociceptive role in inflammation-induced mechanical allodynia, either directly or by conversion to one of its metabolites. Intra-articular injection of carrageenan results in commonly reported swelling of the injured knee and guarding behaviour in all animals [24], but a lack of testosterone during development or in adulthood results in enhanced sensitivity to mechanical stimulation. This organizational effect of testosterone implies that a lack of the hormone during the critical period of sexual differentiation results in disruption of endogenous antinociceptive processes involved in sensitivity to mechanical stimuli following inflammation, and that this alteration of the nervous system is probably permanent.

Gonadal Hormones, Pain and Analgesia

Endogenous opioids, particularly endorphins, interact with gonadal hormones [25–28]. Endogenous or exogenous opioid agonists inhibit the release of luteinizing hormone, which in turn results in decreased secretion of testosterone in males [29]. Many studies have shown important effects of the hypothalamic-pituitary-gonadal axis on the hypothalamic-pituitary-adrenal (HPA) axis. For instance, the fact that oestrogens binding to receptors on the corticoptropin-releasing hormone (CRH) gene can increase CRH activity [30] provides a potential link between the HPA response to stress and female sex hormones. In addition, the presence of oestrogen-receptor-α immunoreactivity in adrenal medullary cells of females [31] supports the suggestion that the female sex steroid, oestrogen, acts directly on the adrenal medulla to induce sympathoadrenal-dependent effects.

It has been reported that cortisol negative feedback could be deranged in patients with fibromyalgia [32]. As previously found in athletes, this altered functioning of the stress response system could be related to down-regulation of glucocorticoid receptors (GcR). In this connection, we observed a significant increase in GcR mRNA expression in patients with fibromyalgia symptoms after a 3-week multi-disciplinary treatment programme including aerobic exercise, physiotherapy and cognitive behavioural therapy [33]. At the same time, the number of tender points, percentage area of pain and actual pain sensation were significantly reduced. These findings suggest that partial relief of muscle pain in FMS patients could be related to better functioning of the stress response system.

Androgens, Pain and Analgesia

Androgens, especially testosterone, are increasingly considered to be important in the modulation of pain mechanisms. In particular, testosterone seems to have a protective role in inflammation. Research on rheumatoid arthritis indicates that androgens protect against inflammation-induced cartilage responses and immunoreactivity (for a review, see [34]). Women with rheumatoid arthritis report pain relief and general improvement of well-being following long-term testosterone administration [35]. Both men and women with rheumatoid arthritis exhibit lower serum testosterone levels than healthy adults [36]. Testosterone has also been used successfully in the treatment of episodic cluster headaches in men [37].

Other studies using inflammatory agents (mainly formalin) to study hormonal influences on nociception have produced conflicting results, but most are in agreement with the suggestion that testosterone plays an antinociceptive role in pain [38–41]. Using a model of repeated painful stimulation, we showed that male rats with physiological levels of testosterone recover better than gonadectomized males [42]; moreover, when supraphysiological levels of testosterone are administered to both male and female rats, there is a reduction in licking duration only in females. Interestingly, this decrease is not present in the flexing or jerking response [43]. Thus, we concluded that a high level of testosterone does not block the nociceptive input (jerking and flexing are unchanged) but induces in females a 'male-like' licking response, the most complex formalin-induced reflex response. These results also suggest that the lower licking levels in males could be kept low by testosterone and that females are sensitive to the testosterone-mediated inhibitory action. This hormone can act directly through the androgen receptors present in many areas of the female CNS.

Oestrogen, pain and analgesia

The presence of oestrogen-sensitive neurons in the superficial dorsal horn lamina of the spinal cord suggests a mechanism by which changing levels of oestrogen can regulate (decrease) pain sensitivity, also through its involvement in the transcriptional control of opioid synthesis and of μ and κ receptors [44]. For instance, the distribution of ER-containing cells in lamina II corresponds to the preferential localization in the spinal cord of pre-proenkephalin-expressing neurons [45].

Simulation of pregnancy plasma levels of oestrogens and progesterone in non-pregnant ovariectomized rats results in an increased pain threshold [46]. Interestingly, this effect is also present in males [47]. We demonstrated that male rats injected intracerebroventricularly with estradiol for 2 days show higher levels of formalin-induced licking than rats receiving saline; in fact, they reach levels previously found in females [48].

On the other hand, it was recently shown that the increased responses of nucleus gracilis neurons during the afternoon of proestrus [49] are partly based on contemporaneous increases in oestrogen levels, possibly acting on dorsal root ganglion cells, whose ER also increase with oestrogen replacement.

Conclusions

The role of gonadal hormones in pain is clearly confirmed by the many studies showing their involvement in pain modulation. An important aspect that needs to be studied more extensively is their role during development. The long-term effects of changes in gonadal hormones due to pharmacological or environmental factors must be taken into account. These hormones should be measured more regularly, and if abnormal levels are found the possibility of hormone replacement therapy should be considered, as commonly occurs for many other circulating hormones.

References

1. Fillingim RB, Edwards RR, Powell T (1999) The relationship of sex and clinical pain to experimental pain responses. Pain 83:419–425
2. Fillingim RB, Ness T (2000) Sex-related hormonal influences on pain and analgesic responses. Neurosci Biobehav Rev 24:485–501
3. Edwards RR, Doleys DM, Lowery D, Fillingim RB (2003) Pain tolerance as a predictor of outcome following multidisciplinary treatment for chronic pain: differential effects as a function of sex. Pain 106:419–426
4. Aloisi AM (2003) Gonadal hormones and sex differences in pain reactivity. Clin J Pain 19:168–174
5. Craft RM (2003) Sex differences in opioid analgesia: "from mouse to man". Clin J Pain 19:175–186
6. Unruh AM (1996) Gender variations in clinical pain experience. Pain 65:123–167
7. Crofford LJ (1998) Neuroendocrine abnormalities in fibromyalgia and related disorders. Am J Med Sci 315:359–366
8. Sandroni P, Benrud-Larson LM, McClelland RL, Low PA (2003) Complex regional pain syndrome type I: incidence and prevalence in Olmsted County: a population-based study. Pain 103:199–207

9. Alamanos Y, Drosos AA (2005) Epidemiology of adult rheumatoid arthritis. Autoimmun Rev 4:130–136
10. Kepler KL, Kest B, Kiefel JM et al (1989) Roles of gender, gonadectomy and estrous phase in the analgesic effects of intracerebroventricular morphine in rats. Pharmacol Biochem Behav 34:119–127
11. Islam AK, Cooper ML Bodnar RJ (1993) Interactions among aging, gender and gonadectomy effects upon morphine antinociception in rats. Physiol Behav 54:45–54
12. Cicero TJ, Nock B, Meyer ER (1996) Gender-related differences in the antinociceptive properties of morphine. J Pharmacol Exp Ther 279:767–773
13. Craft RM, Stratmann JA, Bartok RE (1999) Sex differences in development of morphine tolerance and dependence in the rat. Psychopharmacology 143:1–7
14. Mogil JS, Sternberg WF, Kest B et al (1993) Sex differences in the antagonism of swim stress-induced analgesia: effects of gonadectomy and estrogen replacement. Pain 53:17–25
15. Sternberg WF, Mogil JS, Kest B et al (1995) Neonatal testosterone exposure influences neurochemistry of non-opioid swim stress-induced analgesia in adult mice. Pain 63:321–326
16. Cicero TJ, Nock B, O'Connor L, Meyer ER (2002) Role of steroids in sex differences in morphine-induced analgesia: activational and organizational effects. J Pharmacol Exp Ther 300:695–701
17. McAbee MD, DonCarlos LL (1998) Ontogeny of region-specific sex differences in androgen receptor messenger ribonucleic acid expression in the rat forebrain. Endocrinology 139:1738–1745
18. Yu WH, McGinnis MY (2001) Androgen receptors in cranial nerve motor nuclei of male and female rat. J Neurobiol 46:1–10
19. Kujawa KA, Emeric E, Jones KJ (1991) Testosterone differentially regulates the regenerative properties of injured hamster facial motoneurons. J Neurosci 11:3898–3906
20. Jordan CL, Price Jr, RH Handa RJ (2002) Androgen receptor messenger RNA and protein in adult rat sciatic nerve: implications for site of androgen action. J Neurosci Res 69:509–518
21. McEwen BS (1999) Permanence of brain sex differences and structural plasticity of the adult brain. Proc Natl Acad Sci U S A 96:7128–7130
22. LaCroix-Fralish ML, Tawfik VL, DeLeo JA (2005) The organizational and activational effects of sex hormones on tactile and thermal hypersensitivity following lumbar nerve root injury in male and female rats. Pain 114:71–80
23. Borzan J, Fuchs PN (2006) Organizational and activational effects of testosterone on carrageenan-induced inflammatory pain and morphine analgesia. Neuroscience 143:885–893
24. LaBuda CJ, Fuchs PN (2001) A comparison of chronic aspartame exposure to aspirin on inflammation, hyperalgesia and open field activity following carrageenan-induced monoarthritis. Life Sci 69:443–454
25. Van Vugt DA, Meites J (1980) Influence of endogenous opiates on anterior pituitary function. Fed Proc 39:2533–2538
26. Bhanot B, Wilkinson M (1984) The inhibitory effect of opiates on gonadotrophin secretion is dependent upon gonadal steroids. J Endocrinol 102:133–141
27. Gabriel SM, Berglund LA, Kalra SP et al (1986) The influence of chronic morphine treatment on the negative feedback regulation of gonadotropin secretion by gonadal steroids. Endocrinology 119:2762–2767
28. Kalra PS, Sahu A, Kalra SP (1988) Opiate-induced hypersensitivity to testosterone feedback: pituitary involvement. Endocrinology 122:997–1003
29. Adams ML, Sewing B, Forman JB et al (1993) Opioid-induced suppression of rat testicular function. J Pharmacol Exp Ther 266:323–332
30. Vamvakopoulos NC, Chrousos GP (1993) Evidence of direct estrogenic regulation of human corticotropin-releasing hormone gene expression: potential implications for the sexual dimorphism of the stress response and immune/inflammatory reaction. J Clin Invest 92:1896–1902
31. Saunders PT, Maguire SM, Gaughan J, Millar MR (1997) Expression of oestrogen receptor beta (ER beta) in multiple rat tissues visualised by immunohistochemistry. J Endocrinol 154:R13–R16

32. Lentjes EG, Griep EN, Boersma LW et al (1997) Glucocorticoid receptors, fibromyalgia and low back pain. Psychoneuroendocrinology 22:603–614
33. Bonifazi M, Suman A, Cambiaggi C et al (2006) Changes in salivary cortisol and corticosteroid receptor-alpha mRNA expression following a 3-week multidisciplinary treatment program in patients with fibromyalgia. Psychoneuroendocrinology 31:1076–1086
34. Cutolo M, Sulli A, Capellino S et al (2004) Sex hormones influence on the immune system: basic and clinical aspects in autoimmunity. Lupus 13:635–638
35. Booji A, Biewenga-Booji CM, Huber-Bruning O et al (1996) Androgens as adjuvant treatment in postmenopausal female patients with rheumatoid arthritis. Ann Rheum Dis 55:811–881
36. Straub RH, Cutolo M (2001) Involvement of the hypothalamic-pituitary-adrenal/gonadal axis and the peripheral nervous system in rheumatoid arthritis: viewpoint based on a systemic pathogenetic role. Arthritis Rheum 44:493–507
37. Klimek A (1985) Use of testosterone in the treatment of cluster headache. Eur Neurol 24:53–56
38. Nayebi AR, Ahmadiani (1999) Involvement of the spinal serotonergic system in analgesia produced by castration. Pharmacol Biochem Behav 64:467–471
39. Dina OA, Aley KO, Isenberg W et al (2001) Sex hormones regulate the contribution of PKCε and PKA signaling in inflammatory pain in the rat. Eur J Neurosci 13:2227–2233
40. Gaumond I, Arsenault P, Marchand S (2002) The role of sex hormones on formalin-induced nociceptive responses. Brain Res 958:139–145
41. Butkevich IP, Vershinina EA (2003) Maternal stress differently alters nociceptive behaviors in the formalin test in adult female and male rats. Brain Res 961:159–165
42. Ceccarelli I, Scaramuzzino C, Massafra C, Aloisi AM (2003) The behavioral and neuronal effects induced by repetitive nociceptive stimulation are affected by gonadal hormones in male rats. Pain 104:35–47
43. Aloisi AM, Ceccarelli I, Fiorenzani P et al (2004) Testosterone affects pain-related responses differently in male and female rats. Neurosci Lett 361:262–264
44. Amandusson A, Hallbeck M, Hallbeck AL et al (1999) Estrogen-induced alterations of spinal cord enkephalin gene expression. Pain 83:243–248
45. Amandusson A, Hermanson O, Blomqvist A (1995) Estrogen receptor-like immunoreactivity in the medullary and spinal dorsal horn of the female rat. Neurosci Lett 196:25–28
46. Dawson-Basoa M, Gintzler AR (1998) Gestational and ovarian sex steroid antinociception: synergy between spinal kappa and delta opioid systems. Brain Res 794:61–67
47. Liu NJ, Gintzler AR (2000) Prolonged ovarian sex steroid treatment of male rats produces antinociception: identification of sex-based divergent analgesic mechanisms. Pain 85:273–281
48. Aloisi AM, Ceccarelli I (2000) Role of gonadal hormones in formalin-induced pain responses of male rats: modulation by estradiol and naloxone administration. Neuroscience 95:559–566
49. Bradshaw HB, Berkley K (2000) Estrous changes in responses of rat gracile nucleus neurons to stimulation of skin and pelvic viscera. J Neurosci 20:7722–7772

Chapter 2
Stress and Pregnancy:
CRF as Biochemical Marker

P. Florio, F.M. Reis, S. Luisi, M. De Bonis, I. Zerbetto, R. Battista, M. Quadrifoglio, C. Ferretti, A. Dell'Anna, M. Palumbo and F. Petraglia

Introduction

The initiation, maintenance and termination of pregnancy are related to placental functions, as the human placenta contributes to maintaining equilibrium between the fetus and the mother and regulating the bodily functions of both organisms in a complementary way. This is made possible through the secretion of several growth factors, neurohormones and cytokines by human placenta [1–3].

Among these placental hormones, human placenta, decidua, chorion and amnion produce corticotropin-releasing factor (CRF) [4], the well-known hypothalamic peptide involved in the endocrine adaptations of the hypothalamus-pituitary-adrenal (HPA) axis in response to stress stimuli [5, 6]. This chapter will review experimental and clinical studies showing the role of CRF in physiological (parturition, life and work stress events) and pathological stress conditions (preterm labor, intrauterine infection, hypertensive disorders of pregnancy) occurring during gestation.

CRF-Related Peptides

CRF is a 41-amino-acid peptide released from the median eminence of the hypothalamus, acting at the corticotrophs in the anterior pituitary to stimulate the release of ACTH and related peptides in response to stress events, and modulating behavioral, vascular and immune response to stress [5, 6]. Urocortin is another component of the CRF family, and its sequence is similar to fish urotensin (63%) and human CRF (45%) [7]. As CRF, its addition to cultured pituitary cells stimulates the release of ACTH in a dose-dependent manner [7], indicating that a common signaling pathway exists for both CRF and urocortin.

CRF and urocortin interact with two distinct receptors: R_1 (classified into $R_{1\alpha}$, $R_{1\beta}$, $R_{1\gamma}$ and $R_{1\delta}$ subtypes) and R_2 ($R_{2\alpha}$, $R_{2\beta}$ and $R_{2\gamma}$ subtypes) [8, 9]. Urocortin binds to CRF receptors of types 1 and 2, with a particularly high affinity for the type 2 receptor [7, 10].

CRF-binding protein (CRF-BP), a 37-kDa protein of 322 amino acids, mainly produced by the human brain and the liver [11], is another of the CRF-related peptides. It has been demonstrated that CRF-BP is able to bind circulating CRF and urocortin, thus modulating their actions on pituitary gland [12, 13] by preventing their binding to their own receptors.

Location in Gestational Tissues

CRF, urocortin, CRF-BP and receptors are expressed in human placenta, decidua and fetal membranes. Immunohistochemical studies have demonstrated that CRF is located in cytotrophoblast cells, with a more intense CRF signal in syncytiotrophoblast [3, 14, 15]. Cytotrophoblast cells are transformed into syncytial cells, which release CRF when maintained in culture [3, 16–18].

Placental and decidual cells collected at 8–11 weeks or 38–40 weeks of gestation express urocortin mRNA, and immunohistochemical investigations localized urocortin staining in syncytial cells of trophoblast as well as in amnion, chorion, and decidua of fetal membranes [19, 20], but the urocortin mRNA expression in human placenta does not change throughout gestation [20]. Fluorescent in situ hybridization and immunofluorescence studies demonstrated that syncytiotrophoblast cells and amniotic epithelium are the cell types expressing CRF-R$_{1\alpha}$, CRF-R$_c$ [21], and CRF-R$_{2\beta}$ mRNA [22].

CRF receptors (mRNA and protein) have been also described in human myometrium [23, 24] and endometrium. In particular, pregnant human myometrium expresses the subtypes 1α, 1β, 2α, and 2β and the Rc variant, whereas only the 1α, 1β, and 2β receptors are detectable in nonpregnant myometrium [24] and endometrium [11, 25, 26].

In Vitro Effects

In nonpregnant women, the close relationship between catecholamines, HPA axis and stress events represents a classic finding of neuroendocrinology [27], given that increased production of catecholamines and CRF characterizes the adaptive responses to stressful events [28]. Placental ACTH is a product of the propiomelanocortin (POMC) gene and has the same structure of pituitary ACTH, retaining its immunogenic and biologic activity [29, 30]. Placental ACTH is localized to the cytotrophoblast in the first trimester and to the syncytiotrophoblast in the second and third trimesters [31].

Placental Hormonogenesis

The addiction of CRF and urocortin stimulates placental ACTH release. The effect is mediated by CRF receptors, as the co-incubation of cultured placenta cells with specific CRF receptor antagonists inhibits the release of ACTH induced by CRF and urocortin. Furthermore, the addition of CRF-BP reverses the effects of CRF on ACTH in human placenta. Indeed, CRF-BP binds CRF in vitro with great affinity: on a perfused pituitary cell column system the bioactivity of CRF is reduced by co-incubation with CRF-BP [32], whereas in vivo the presence of the binding protein shortens the half-life of immunoreactive CRF [33, 34] (Fig. 1).

CRF, urocortin and ACTH stimulate the release of PGF_{2a} and PGE_2 from cultured amnion, chorion, decidual and placental tissues [35–37], and these effects are inhibited in the presence of specific antisera to CRF and to ACTH. In placenta, but not in amnion or decidua, the stimulatory effect of CRF on PGF_{2a} and PGE_2 output is attenuated in the presence of an antibody to ACTH, thus supporting the possibility of paracrine stimulation by CRF and ACTH of prostaglandin production in intrauterine tissues [38]. Urocortin has CRF-like effects on placental cells and tissue explants, because it stimulates ACTH and prostaglandin secretion [35, 39]. CRF markedly stimulates the release of immunoreactive oxytocin from cultured placental cells in a dose-dependent fashion [40].

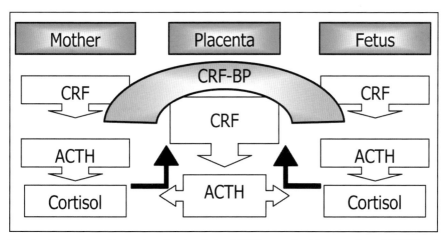

Fig. 1 Placental corticotropin-releasing factor (CRF) may affect the secretion of ACTH and cortisol from the mother and the fetus. The effects are counteracted by CRF-binding protein (CRF-BP)

Blood Flow Regulation

Several in vitro experiments have demonstrated that CRF has vasodilatory effects in the human fetal-placental circulation. The effects are mediated by nitric oxide (NO) and by cyclic GMP, as blocking the synthesis of these molecules causes marked attenuation of CRF-stimulated vasodilatation [41]. The addition of CRF to preconstricted placental vessels is able to attenuate all constrictor mechanisms without variation in CRF potency as a vasodilator agent. CRF-induced vasodilatation appears to be mediated by a CRF receptor, as the vasodilatory response to CRF is antagonized in the presence of CRF receptor antagonists [42, 43]. CRF-induced vasodilatation occurred at concentrations comparable to plasma CRF levels found in the maternal and fetal circulations [44], and CRF is approximately 50 times more potent than prostacyclin as a vasodilator agent [42, 43].

Urocortin has the same effects as CRF: administered intravenously in rats, it is more potent than CRF in causing hypotension [7, 45] and, with respect to placental circulation, it causes vasodilatation, reducing fetal-placental vascular resistance via CRF type 2 receptors, and being more potent than CRF [46]. As the fetal vessels of the human placenta are not innervated, control of blood flow in this vascular bed is partly dependent on locally produced and circulating vasoactive factors [47]. As syncytiotrophoblast is the main source of CRF during pregnancy [44, 48, 49], placental CRF may access the fetal-placental circulation to cause dilatation by paracrine or endocrine mechanisms. It may be released locally to affect the vascular smooth muscle and endothelium, or it may be secreted into the fetal-placental circulation and travel to its site of action through the placental vascular system.

Myometrial Contractility

The family of CRF-related peptides is suggested to play important roles in the control of myometrial contractility during pregnancy and labor [50]. Recent data highlight the role played by CRF in myometrial contractility, based on the fact that CRF mediates its actions on human myometrium through the activation of two distinct classes of CRF receptor, R_1 and R_2 [51]. Contrasting data exist on the net role played by CRF, some suggesting CRF as an important uterotonic [52, 53], others indicating it as the main uterine quiescence factor [51, 54] to prevent uterine contractions during pregnancy. In addition, different myometrial CRF receptors are recruited at labor, and this recruitment is dynamically and differentially modulated by the great hormonal changes occurring at term pregnancy, so that CRF actions in vivo may differ from actions reported in vitro, according to differences in myometrial CRF receptor expression and the induced affinity-state [55]. In fact, in vitro CRF and urocortin directly enhance prostaglandin-induced myometrial contractility, and the effect is counteracted by CRF receptor antagonists and by CRF-BP.

Urocortin, more than CRF, is able to induce different intracellular signals involved in the regulation of myometrial contractility [50]. Robinson et al. [56] suggested that placental CRF may also stimulate fetal pituitary ACTH, which triggers secretion of fetal adrenal dehydroepiandrosterone sulfate (DHEAS), which in turn is used by the placenta for conversion to estrogen by the process of aromatization [57]. This increase in estrogen then could serve as a trigger for the cascade of events leading to labor and parturition. In fact, estrogens increase uterine contractility by increasing myometrial excitability, myometrial responsiveness to oxytocin and other uterotonic agents, as well as stimulating the synthesis and release of prostaglandins by fetal membranes [57]. Furthermore, estrogens stimulate proteolytic enzymes in the cervix, such as collagenase, which break down the extracellular matrix, permitting the cervix to dilate.

Secretion in Biological Fluids

From intrauterine tissues, CRF is released into the maternal and umbilical cord plasma as well as the amniotic fluid. Plasma CRF levels are low in nonpregnant women (less than 10 pg/ml) and become higher during the first trimester of pregnancy, rising steadily until term [58–60]. CRF is also measurable in fetal circulation, and a linear correlation exists between maternal and fetal plasma CRF levels, despite umbilical cord plasma CRF levels being 20 to 30 times lower than in maternal circulation [61].

CRF-BP is measurable in maternal plasma, and levels remain stable in nonpregnant women and during gestation until the third trimester of pregnancy [11, 62]. The existence of a binding protein for CRF explains why there is not a dramatic increase of ACTH despite high levels of CRF during the third trimester of pregnancy [63, 64]. In fact, it was confirmed that most of the endogenous CRF in both maternal plasma [18] and amniotic fluid [62] is carrier-bound and therefore has reduced bioactivity.

Maternal plasma CRF-BP concentrations decrease markedly in the last 4–6 weeks before labor [11, 64, 65], returning to approximately nonpregnant levels during the first 24 h post partum. Thus, opposite changes in concentrations of CRF (higher) and CRF-BP (lower) in maternal plasma occur at term, so that the availability of bioactive CRF increases during the activation of labor.

Labor and Delivery

Several pieces of evidence support the link between placental CRF and the stress of parturition in humans. During spontaneous labor, maternal plasma CRF levels rise progressively, reaching the maximum values at the most advanced stages of cervical dilatation [63, 66, 67]. In addition, individuals who undergo elective cesarean delivery have plasma and amniotic fluid CRF levels significantly lower than those who have had spontaneous vaginal delivery [68]. The amount of CRF in placental extracts obtained at term after spontaneous vaginal delivery is significantly greater than the amount extracted from placentas obtained after caesarean delivery [68]. By contrast, during spontaneous physiological labor a significant decrease has been observed in CRF-BP levels in maternal plasma [63, 68], cord blood [68] and amniotic fluid [69].

With respect to urocortin, maternal levels at labor were higher than those previously reported during pregnancy, but they did not change significantly at the different stages of labor when evaluated longitudinally. Some mothers displayed a trend towards increasing levels, whilst others had variable concentrations [70].

Preterm Labor

Preterm birth is a major complication of pregnancy and remains a leading cause of neonatal morbidity and mortality worldwide. Women with preterm labor have maternal plasma CRF levels significantly higher than those measured in the course of normal pregnancy (Fig. 2) [71]. This finding suggests that the increase in CRF levels in women with preterm labor is not due to the process of labor itself, but may indeed be part of the mechanism controlling the onset of labor. The continued elevation of CRF preceding clinical evidence of uterine contraction suggests that CRF secretion is not sufficient to induce initiation of labor, and other factors are required in this event [68].

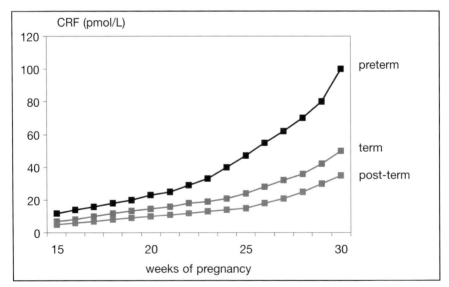

Fig. 2 Changes of maternal plasma CRF levels during pregnancies that ended in term, preterm and post-term deliveries

Maternal plasma CRF is higher in women with threatened preterm labor who give birth within 24 h from admission compared with those delivered after 24 h or with normal pregnant women at the same stage of gestation. This difference was observed at 28–32 weeks' and at 32–36 weeks' gestation, but not before 28 weeks [60]. Maternal and fetal plasma CRF-BP levels are low in preterm labor [72, 73], resembling the physiological pattern observed at term. Because CRF-BP modulates the CRF-induced ACTH and prostaglandin release from decidual cells as well as the myometrial contractility activated by CRF [42], the precocious fall in CRF-BP levels may be involved in the pathophysiology of preterm labor. Finally, recent evidence further suggested that elevated levels of CRF are linked to preterm labor and delivery, but also that CRF is only one of several systems involved in this process [74, 75].

Chorionamnionitis

During pregnancy, the secretion of CRF from intrauterine sources is autonomous, but increasing evidence indicates that maternal and/or fetal physiological and patho-logical stress conditions may influence this function [76, 77]. Intrauterine infection is a stress situation associated with a significant CRF elevation in placental extracts, maternal plasma and amniotic fluid [37]. In addition, we found that women with intrauterine infection (i.e. microbial invasion of the amniotic cavity) had significantly higher amniotic fluid and umbilical cord plasma CRF and CRF-BP levels, but unchanged levels of ACTH and cortisol concentrations [78]. However, it is well known that CRF triggers ACTH and cortisol secretion [79]. The increased levels of CRF-BP in cases of maternal infection may prevent the CRF-induced stimulation of ACTH and cortisol, even in the presence of high CRF concentrations in amni-otic fluid and umbilical cord plasma.

A possible explanation for these increases may be found in the genomic char-acterization of CRF-BP, which has revealed acute phase response elements. One of them is known to bind the transcription factor NF- B, which regulates immunoglob-ulin and interleukin transcription, and is thought to play a role in the response to inflammation [11, 80]. On the other hand, cytokines stimulate CRF expression and secretion [81, 82], so the increased levels of CRF-BP in the presence of intrauter-ine infection may play a role in regulating inflammatory responses evoked by CRF.

Preeclampsia and Fetal Growth Restriction

Preeclampsia affects 10–12% of pregnancies, requires intense monitoring and clin-ical supervision, and is potentially threatening to mother and fetus [83, 84]. Preeclampsia is associated with abnormal placentation, due to altered cytotrophoblast proliferation and invasion of endometrium, causing reduced placental perfusion and impairment of placental angiogenesis, with insufficiency and failure of remodeling of the spiral arteries [85]. Trophoblastic abnormalities play a role in the development of preeclampsia, and alterations in the secretion of placental hormones and/or factors may be considered manifestations of the earlier stages of the disease, in addition to uteroplacental and fetal blood flow alterations (evaluated by Doppler velocimetry). These modifications reduce the transport of oxygen and substrates from the mother to the fetus through the human placenta, and therefore fetal growth restriction is often associated with preeclampsia [86].

CRF levels are elevated in the fetal and maternal circulation in these abnormal pregnancies. In patients with pregnancy-induced hypertension (PIH), maternal CRF levels at all stages of pregnancy are significantly higher than in healthy controls [87–89]. Moreover, maternal concentrations of CRF are greatly increased in preeclampsia [76, 90] in the presence of plasma CRF-BP levels significantly lower than those in healthy controls [91]. In addition, cord venous plasma CRF concentrations are significantly higher in patients with preeclampsia and higher than those in cord arterial plasma, indicating secretion of CRF from the placenta into the fetal circulation [90]. In addition to CRF, other hormones with vasodilatory actions and involved in the stress response such as ACTH and cortisol are increased in fetuses from normotensive pregnancies [92] as well as in those with fetal growth restriction [83, 93, 94].

Concentrations of CRF in fetal circulation are significantly increased in pregnancies complicated by abnormal umbilical artery flow velocity waveforms, thus representing a stress-responsive compensatory mechanism in the human placenta [95]. It is not known whether this deranged secretion is part of the primary pathophysiology of these conditions or occurs as a secondary response to the increased vascular resistance in abnormal pregnancies.

Conclusions

In the event of stressful conditions, such as reduced placental blood flow, chronic hypoxia or infection, the human placenta responds with increased CRF and urocortin secretion, with the aim of dilating the placental circulation, facilitating oxygen and substrate availability, facilitating term and preterm labor, and also preparing the fetus for birth, increasing cortisol secretion for lung maturation. Thus, the placental release of CRF as a stress factor is the final pathway triggered by the human placenta to help the mother and the fetus to escape a hostile environment.

Thus, in a scenario of maternal and/or fetal stress elicited by a number of pathological conditions, placental CRF and CRF-related peptides appear to play a role in coordinating the adaptive changes to promote uterine perfusion, maternal metabolism, fluid balance and, possibly, uterine contractility.

References

1. Petraglia F, Volpe A, Genazzani AR et al (1990) Neuroendocrinology of the human placenta. Front Neuroendocrinol 11:6–37
2. Reis FM, Florio P, Cobellis L et al (2001) Human placenta as a source of neuroendocrine factors. Biol Neonate 79:150–156
3. Petraglia F, Sawchenko PE, Rivier J, Vale W (1987) Evidence for local stimulation of ACTH secretion by corticotropin-releasing factor in human placenta. Nature 328:717–719
4. Petraglia F, Tabanelli S, Galassi MC et al (1992) Human decidua and in vitro decidualized endometrial stromal cells at term contain immunoreactive corticotropin-releasing factor (CRF) and CRF messenger ribonucleic acid. J Clin Endocrinol Metab 74:1427–1431
5. Vale W, Rivier C, Brown MR et al (1983) Chemical and biological characterization of corticotropin releasing factor. Recent Prog Horm Res 39:245–270
6. Orth DN (1992) Corticotropin-releasing hormone in humans. Endocr Rev 13:164–191
7. Vaughan J, Donaldson C, Bittencourt J et al (1995) Urocortin, a mammalian neuropeptide related to fish urotensin I and to corticotropin-releasing factor. Nature 378:287–292
8. Liaw CW, Lovenmerg TW, Barry G et al (1996) Cloning and characterization of the human corticotropin-releasing factor-2 receptor complementary deoxyribonucleic acid. Endocrinology 137:72–77
9. Valdenaire O, Giller T, Breu V et al (1997) A new functional isoform of the human CRF2 receptor for corticotropin-releasing factor. Biochim Biophys Acta 1352:129–132
10. Chen R, Lewis K, Perrin MH, Vale W (1993) Expression and cloning of a human corticotropin-releasing factor receptor. Proc Natl Acad Sci U S A 90:8967–8971
11. Petraglia F, Florio P, Gallo R et al (1996) Corticotropin-releasing factor-binding protein: origins and possible functions. Horm Res 45:187–191
12. Potter E, Behan DP, Fischer WH et al (1991) Cloning and characterization of the cDNAs for human and rat corticotropin releasing factor-binding proteins. Nature 349:423–426
13. Potter E, Behan DP, Linton EA et al (1992) The central distribution of a corticotropin-releasing factor (CRF)-binding protein predicts multiple sites and modes of interaction with CRF. Proc Natl Acad Sci U S A 89:4192–4196
14. Saijonmaa X, Laatikainen T, Wahlstrom T (1988) Corticotropin releasing factor in human placenta: localization, concentration and release in vitro. Placenta 9:373–385
15. Riley SC, Walton JC, Herlick JM, Challis JR (1991) The localization and distribution of corticotropin-releasing hormone in the human placenta and fetal membranes throughout gestation. J Clin Endocrinol Metab 72:1001–1007
16. Frim DM, Emanuel RL, Robinson BG et al (1988) Characterization and gestational regulation of corticotropin-releasing hormone messenger RNA in human placenta. J Clin Invest 82:287–292
17. Jones SA, Brooks AN, Challis JR (1989) Steroids modulate corticotropin-releasing hormone production in human fetal membranes and placenta. J Clin Endocrinol Metab 68:825–830
18. Riley SC, Challis JR (1991) Corticotropin-releasing hormone production by the placenta and fetal membranes. Placenta 12:105–119
19. Petraglia F, Florio P, Gallo R et al (1996) Human placenta and fetal membranes express human urocortin mRNA and peptide. J Clin Endocrinol Metab 81:3807–3810
20. Florio P, Rivest S, Reis FM et al (1999) Lack of gestational-related changes of urocortin gene expression in human placenta. Prenat Neonat Med 4:296–300
21. Karteris E, Grammatopoulos D, Dai Y et al (1998) The human placenta and fetal membranes express the corticotropin-releasing hormone receptor 1α (CRH-1α) and the CRH-C variant receptor. J Clin Endocrinol Metab 83:1376–1379
22. Florio P, Franchini A, Reis FM et al (2000) Human placenta, chorion, amnion and decidua express different variants of corticotropin-releasing factor receptor messenger RNA. Placenta 21:32–37
23. Rodrýguez-Linares B, Linton EA, Phaneuf S (1998) Expression of corticotropin releasing hormone (CRH) receptor mRNA and protein in the human myometrium. J Endocrinol 156:15–21

24. Grammatopoulos D, Dai Y, Chen J et al (1998) Human corticotropin-releasing hormone receptor: differences in subtype expression between pregnant and nonpregnant myometria. J Clin Endocrinol Metab 83:2539–2544
25. Di Blasio AM, Giraldi FP, Vigano P et al (1997) Expression of corticotropin-releasing hormone and its R1 receptor in human endometrial stromal cells. J Clin Endocrinol Metab 82:1594–1597
26. Petraglia F, Potter E, Cameron VA et al (1993) Corticotropin-releasing factor-binding protein is produced by human placenta and intrauterine tissues. J Clin Endocrinol Metab 77:919–924
27. Chrousos GP (1998) Editorial: ultradian, circadian, and stress-related hypothalamic-pituitary-adrenal axis activity – a dynamic digital-to-analog modulation. Endocrinology 139:437–440
28. Chrousos GP, Gold PW (1992) The concepts of stress and stress system disorders: overview of physical and behavioral homeostasis. JAMA 267:1252
29. Waddell BJ, Burton PJ (1993) Release of bioactive ACTH by perifused human placenta at early and late gestation. J Endocrinol 136:345–353
30. Smith R, Thomson M (1991) Neuroendocrinology of the hypothalamo-pituitary-adrenal axis in pregnancy and the puerperium. Baillieres Clin Endocrinol Metab 5:167–186
31. Cooper ES, Greer IA, Brooks AN (1996) Placental proopiomelanocortin gene expression, adrenocorticotropin tissue concentrations, and immunostaining increase throughout gestation and are unaffected by prostaglandins, antiprogestins, or labor. J Clin Endocrinol Metab 81:4462–4469
32. Woods RJ, Kennedy KM, Gibbins JM et al (1994) Corticotropin releasing factor binding protein dimerizes after association with ligand. Endocrinology 135:768–773
33. Petraglia F, Florio P, Gallo R et al (1996) Corticotropin-releasing factor-binding protein: origins and possible functions. Horm Res 45:187–191
34. Woods RJ, Grossman A, Saphier P et al (1994) Association of human corticotropin-releasing hormone to its binding protein in blood may trigger clerance of the complex. J Clin Endocrinol Metab 78:73–76
35. Petraglia F, Florio P, Benedetto C et al (1999) Urocortin stimulates placental adrenocorticotropin and prostaglandin release and myometrial contractility in vitro. J Clin Endocrinol Metab 84:1420–1423
36. Jones SA, Challis JR (1989) Local stimulation of prostaglandin production by corticotropin-releasing hormone in human fetal membranes and placenta. Biochem Biophys Res Commun 159:192–199
37. Petraglia F, Benedetto C, Florio P et al (1995) Effect of corticotropin-releasing factor-binding protein on prostaglandin release from cultured maternal decidua and on contractile activity of human myometrium in vitro. J Clin Endocrinol Metab 80:3073–3076
38. Jones SA, Challis JR (1990) Effects of corticotropin-releasing hormone and adrenocorticotropin on prostaglandin output by human placenta and fetal membranes. Gynecol Obstet Invest 29:165–168
39. Leitch IM, Boura AL, Botti C et al (1998) Vasodilator actions of urocortin and related peptides in the human perfused placenta in vitro. J Clin Endocrinol Metab 83:4510–4513
40. Florio P, Lombardo M, Gallo R et al (1996) Activin A, corticotropin-releasing factor and prostaglandin F2 alpha increase immunoreactive oxytocin release from cultured human placental cells. Placenta 17:307–311
41. Clifton VL, Read MA, Leitch IM et al (1994) Corticotropin-releasing hormone-induced vasodilatation in the human fetal placental circulation. J Clin Endocrinol Metab 79:666–669
42. Clifton VL, Owens PC, Robinson PJ, Smith R (1995) Identification and characterization of a corticotrophin-releasing hormone receptor in human placenta. Eur J Endocrinol 133:591–597
43. Clifton VL, Read MA, Leitch IM et al (1995) Corticotropin-releasing hormone-induced vasodilatation in the human fetal-placental circulation: involvement of the nitric oxide-cyclic guanosine 3′,5′-monophosphate-mediated pathway. J Clin Endocrinol Metab 80:2888–2893

44. Petraglia F (1996) Endocrine role of the placenta and related membranes. Eur J Endocrinol 135:166–167
45. Torpy DJ, Chrousos GP (1996) The three-way interactions between the hypothalamic-pituitary-adrenal and gonadal axes and the immune system [review]. Baillieres Clin Rheumatol 10:181–198
46. Leitch IM, Boura AL, Botti C et al (1998) Vasodilator actions of urocortin and related peptides in the human perfused placenta in vitro. J Clin Endocrinol Metab 83:4510–4513
47. Boura AL, Walters WA, Read MA, Leitch IM (1994) Autacoids and control of human placental blood flow [review]. Clin Exp Pharmacol Physiol 21:737–748
48. Simoncini T, Apa R, Reis FM et al (1999) Human umbilical vein endothelial cells: a new source and potential target for corticotropin-releasing factor. J Clin Endocrinol Metab 84:2802–2806
49. Challis JR, Sloboda D, Matthews SG et al (2001) The fetal placental hypothalamic-pituitary-adrenal (HPA) axis, parturition and post natal health [review]. Mol Cell Endocrinol 185:135–144
50. Karteris E, Hillhouse EW, Grammatopoulos D (2004) Urocortin II is expressed in human pregnant myometrial cells and regulates myosin light chain phosphorylation: potential role of the type-2 corticotropin-releasing hormone receptor in the control of myometrial contractility. Endocrinology 145:890–900
51. Grammatopoulos DK, Hillhouse EW (1999) Role of corticotropin-releasing hormone in onset of labour. Lancet 354:1546–1549
52. Benedetto C, Petraglia F, Marozio L et al (1994) Corticotropin releasing hormone increases prostaglandin F2a activity on human myometrium. Am J Obstet Gynecol 171:126–31
53. Quartero HW, Fry CH (1989) Placental corticotrophin releasing factor may modulate human parturition. Placenta 10:439–443
54. Quartero HW, Srivatsa G, Gillham B (1992) Role for cyclic adenosine monophosphate in the synergistic interaction between oxytocin and corticotrophin-releasing factor in isolated human gestational myometrium. Clin Endocrinol (Oxf) 36:141–145
55. Hillhouse EW, Grammatopoulos DK (2000) CRH and urocortin actions during human pregnancy and labour. Stress 4:235–246
56. Robinson BG, Emanuel RL, Frim DM, Majzoub JA (1988) Glucocorticoid stimulates expression of corticotropin-releasing hormone gene in human placenta. Proc Natl Acad Sci U S A 85:5244–5348
57. Challis JRG, Matthews SG, Gibb W, Lye SJ (2000) Endocrine and paracrine regulation of birth at term and preterm. Endocr Rev 21:514–550
58. Stalla GK, Bost H, Stalla J (1989) Human corticotropin-releasing hormone during pregnancy. Gynecol Endocrinol 3:1–10
59. Campbell EA, Linton EA, Wolfe CDA et al (1987) Plasma corticotropin releasing hormone concentrations during pregnancy and parturition. J Clin Endocrinol Metab 63:1054–1059
60. Petraglia F, Florio P, Benedetto C et al (1996) High levels of corticotropin-releasing factor (CRF) are inversely correlated with low levels of maternal CRF-binding protein in pregnant women with pregnancy-induced hypertension. J Clin Endocrinol Metab 81:852–856
61. Economides D, Linton E, Nicolaides K et al (1987) Relationship between maternal and fetal corticotrophin-releasing hormone-41 and ACTH levels in human mid-trimester pregnancy. J Endocrinol 114:497–501
62. Suda T, Iwashita M, Sumitomo T et al (1991) Presence of CRH-binding protein in amniotic fluid and in umbilical cord plasma. Acta Endocrinol 125:165–169
63. Linton EA, Wolfe CDA, Behan D, Lowry PJ (1988) A specific carrier substance for human corticotropin releasing factor in late gestational maternal plasma which could mask the ACTH releasing activity. Clin Endocrinol 28:315–324
64. Orth DN, Mount CD (1987) Specific high affinity binding protein for human corticotropin releasing hormone in normal human plasma. Biochem Biophys Res Commun 143:411–417

65. Linton EA, Perkins AV, Woods RJ et al (1993) Corticotropin releasing hormone-binding protein (CRH-BP): plasma levels decrease during the third trimester of normal human pregnancy. J Clin Endocrinol Metab 76:260–262
66. Goland RS, Wardlaw SL, Stark RI et al (1986) High levels of corticotropin-releasing hormone immunoactivity in maternal and fetal plasma during pregnancy. J Clin Endocrinol Metab 63:1199–1203
67. Petraglia F, Giardino L, Coukos G et al (1990) Corticotropin-releasing factor and parturition: plasma and amniotic fluid levels and placental binding sites. Obstet Gynecol 75:784–790
68. McLean M, Bisit A, Davies JJ et al (1995) A placental clock controlling the length of human pregnancy. Nat Med 1:460–463
69. Florio P, Woods RJ, Genazzani AR et al (1997) Changes in amniotic fluid immunoreactive corticotropin-releasing factor (CRF) and CRF-binding protein levels in pregnant women at term and during labor. J Clin Endocrinol Metab 82:835–838
70. Florio P, Cobellis L, Woodman J et al (2002) Levels of maternal plasma corticotropin-releasing factor (CRF) and urocortin at labor. J Soc Gynecol Investig 9:233-237
71. Korebrit C, Ramirez MM, Watson L et al (1998) Maternal corticotropin-releasing hormone is increased with impending preterm birth. J Clin Endocrinol Metab 83:1585–1591
72. Berkowitz GS, Lapinski RH, Lockwood CJ et al (1996) Corticotropin-releasing factor and its binding protein: maternal serum levels in term and preterm deliveries. Am J Obstet Gynecol 174:1477–1483
73. Perkins AV, Eben F, Wolfe CD et al (1993) Plasma measurements of corticotrophin-releasing hormone-binding protein in normal and abnormal human pregnancy. J Endocrinol 138:149–157
74. Erickson K, Thorsen P, Chrousos G et al (2001) Preterm birth: associated neuroendocrine, medical, and behavioral risk factors. J Clin Endocrinol Metab 86, 2544–2552
75. Reis FM, D'Antona D, Petraglia F (2002) Predictive value of hormone measurements in maternal and fetal complications of pregnancy. Endocr Rev 23:230–257
76. Petraglia F, Florio P, Nappi C, Genazzani AR (1996) Peptide signaling in human placenta and membranes: autocrine, paracrine, and endocrine mechanisms. Endocrine Rev 17:156–186
77. Reis FM, Fadalti M, Florio P, Petraglia F (1996) Putative role of placental corticotropin-releasing factor in the mechanisms of human parturition. J Soc Gynecol Invest 6:109–119
78. Florio P, Severi FM, Ciarmela P et al (2002) Placental stress factors and maternal-fetal adaptive response: the corticotropin-releasing factor family. Endocrine 19:91–102
79. Florio P, Petraglia F (2002) Human placental corticotropin-releasing factor (CRF) in the adaptive response to pregnancy. Stress 4:247–261
80. Lowry PJ, Woods RJ, Baigent S (1996) Corticotropin-releasing factor and its binding protein. Pharmacol Biochem Behav 54:305–308
81. Petraglia F, Garuti GC, De Ramundo B et al (1990) Mechanism of action of interleukin-1 beta in increasing corticotropin-releasing factor and adrenocorticotropin hormone release from cultured human placental cells. Am J Obstet Gynecol 163:1307–1312
82. Angioni S, Petraglia F, Gallinelli A et al (1993) Corticotropin-releasing hormone modulates cytokines release in cultured human peripheral blood mononuclear cells. Life Sci 53:1735–1742
83. Redman CWG (1991) Pre-eclampsia and placenta. Placenta 12:301–308
84. Talosi G, Endreffy E, Turi S, Nemeth I (2000) Molecular and genetic aspects of preeclampsia: state of the art. Mol Genet Metab 71:565–572
85. Roberts JM, Cooper DW (2001) Pathogenesis and genetics of pre-eclampsia. Lancet 357:53–6
86. Luckas MJ, Sandland R, Hawe J et al (1998) Fetal growth retardation and second trimester maternal serum human chorionic gonadotrophin levels. Placenta 19:143–147
87. Wolfe CD, Patel SP, Campbell EA et al (1988) Plasma corticotrophin-releasing factor (CRF) in normal pregnancy. Br J Obstet Gynaecol 95:997–1002
88. Wolfe CD, Patel SP, Linton EA et al (1988) Plasma corticotrophin-releasing factor (CRF) in abnormal pregnancy. Br J Obstet Gynaecol 95:1003–1006

89. Jeske W, Soszynski P, Lukaszewicz E et al (1990) Enhancement of plasma corticotropin-releasing hormone in pregnancy-induced hypertension. Acta Endocrinol (Copenh) 122:711–714
90. Laatikainen T, Virtanen T, Kaaja R et al (1991) Corticotropin-releasing hormone in maternal and cord plasma in pre-eclampsia. Eur J Obstet Gynecol Reprod Biol 39:19–24
91. Perkins AV, Linton EA, Eben F et al (1995) Corticotrophin-releasing hormone and corticotrophin-releasing hormone binding protein in normal and pre-eclamptic human pregnancies. Br J Obstet Gynaecol 102:118–122
92. Goland RS, Conwell IM, Jozak S (1995) The effect of pre-eclampsia on human placental corticotrophin-releasing hormone content and processing. Placenta 16:375–382
93. Goland RS, Jozak S, Warren WB et al (1993) Elevated levels of umbilical cord plasma corticotropin-releasing hormone in growth-retarded fetuses. J Clin Endocrinol Metab 77:1174–1179
94. Ahmed I, Glynn BP, Perkins AV et al (2000) Processing of procorticotropin-releasing hormone (pro-CRH): molecular forms of CRH in normal and preeclamptic pregnancy. J Clin Endocrinol Metab 85:755–764
95. Giles W, O'Callaghan S, Read M et al (1997) Placental nitric oxide synthase activity and abnormal umbilical artery flow velocity waveforms. Obstet Gynecol 89:49–52

Chapter 3
Pain Control During Labour

C. Benedetto, M. Zonca, L. Bonino, S. Blefari and E. Gollo

Labour pain is described as a complex, subjective and multidimensional experience characterized by severe pain. Usually, labour is divided into three stages. The *first stage* is defined as the beginning of regular uterine contractions until cervical dilatation is completed. The *second stage* is from the end of the first stage until the delivery of the fetus, and the third stage continues until the placenta and membranes have been discharged. During the *first stage* the pain is mainly visceral and mediated by the T10–L1 segments of the spine, while during the second stage, an additional somatic component is present, mediated by the S1–S4 segments of the spine.

It may be speculated that labour pain involves both maternal and fetal aspects. The increased maternal levels of catecholamines, as a consequence of pain, could lead to detrimental effects on a less well fetus (particularly if there is poor placental function). Catecholamines on the one hand increase maternal heart rate, stroke volume and heart contractility, causing an increase in the myocardial workload and oxygen consumption; on the other hand they also increase peripheral vasoconstriction, causing a decrease in placental perfusion. Moreover, labour pain is associated with hyperventilation, which leads to respiratory alkalosis and ultimately causes metabolic acidosis and fetal hypoxia. The treatment of pain gives relief to the mother and in theory could improve fetal well-being (Fig. 1).

The goals of labour analgesia are to: (1) give good pain relief, (2) be safe for the mother and the fetus/newborn, (3) be easy to manage and adapt for each woman, and (4) have known and predictable effects and not interfere with the dynamics of labour and the motor blockade.

Pain relief during labour can be achieved by *non-pharmacological* and *pharmacological analgesia*. The former includes transcutaneous electrical nerve stimulation (TENS), acupuncture, hydrotherapy, hypnotherapy, massage, movement and positioning, and psychological support; the latter includes analgesia by inhalation, parenteral opioids and locoregional blockade (paracervical, epidural or combined spinal-epidural).

G. Buonocore, C.V. Bellieni (eds), *Neonatal Pain. Suffering, Pain and Risk of Brain Damage in the Fetus and Newborn*, © Springer 2008

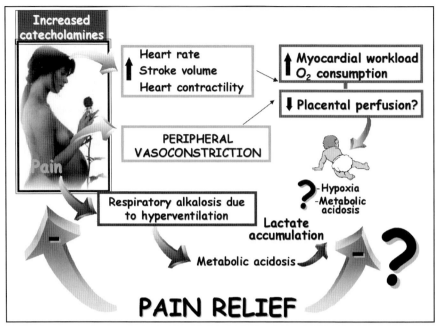

Fig. 1 Hypothetical effect of pain relief on fetal well-being. Labor pain increases maternal catecholamines and causes hyperventilation: both could lead to detrimental effects on less well fetus, such as hypoxya and metabolic acidosis, through the action on the cardiovascular, respiratory and metabolic system. The pain rilief given to the mother may improve fetal well-being

Non-pharmacological Analgesia

Non-pharmacological analgesia can be useful to give relief to the mother. However, the results of the few available controlled trials are contradictory. Further well-designed randomized controlled trials are needed [1].

Pharmacological Analgesia

The *inhalation of a mixture of 50% N_2O/O_2* has no detrimental effects on the mother and the fetus/newborn, but it is no longer used because of its poor efficacy in pain relief.

Parenteral opioids give good pain relief when given in high doses, but can cause respiratory depression, hypotension and a decrease in myometrial contractility in the mother, and severe respiratory depression in the baby [2]. They have hence been used at lower doses, but with limited analgesic effects on labour pain. Fentanyl is the preferred choice in obstetrics because of its short neonatal half-life (5.3 h vs 20–60 h for meperidine).

Epidural analgesia is the most flexible and effective and least depressing on the central nervous system of all other pharmacological techniques. New forms of epidural analgesia use a combination of opioids and local anaesthetics in low doses, instead of traditional techniques, which employ only local anaesthetics. The advantages of adding an opioid during the first stage of labour are that it has greater efficacy on visceral pain, and does not interfere in motor functions, allowing the mother to walk. Maternal motor function during the second stage of labour is also preserved by the use of local anaesthetics such as levobupivacaine and ropivacaine, which selectively block the sensor fibres [2]. Epidural analgesia should be used only during the first stage of labour in order to avoid prolonging labour, and in order not to risk an increase in instrumental deliveries (Table 1).

In our hospital epidural analgesia during labour is widely used: it is employed in 32% of vaginal deliveries. Like other authors, we have observed no significant differences in the rate of caesarean section, and a significant increment in oxytocin augmentation as significant increment in oxigen augmentation between patients receiving epidural analgesia and controls. In contrast with published data, we have not observed an increase in instrumental vaginal deliveres, probably because we used epidural analgesia only during the first stage of labor.

In our experience, the Apgar score is not influenced by epidural analgesia. A meta-analysis by the Cochrane Library did not reveal any effects of epidural analgesia on fetal heart rate, meconium abnormalities or the number of newborns with an Apgar score lower than 7 at 5 min. Neonates of mothers with epidural analgesia had les risk of having a pH below 7.2 in the umbilical artery (Table 1).

Combined spinal-epidural (CSE) analgesia consists in a single intrathecal injection of opioids with or without local anaesthetics plus epidural analgesia. It gives rapid pain relief, minimal motor blockade and faster cervical dilatation, and is associated with more spontaneous deliveries and fewer instrumental deliveries than epidural analgesia. Some authors observed severe fetal bradycardia within 60 min after the administration of spinal fentanyl and an increased risk of caesarean sections because of fetal heart rate abnormalities. However, the Task Force on Obstetrical Anaesthesia and Consultants [3] agree that combined spinal-epidural does not increase the risk of fetal or neonatal complications. The use of labour analgesia (epidural, combined spinal-epidural) does not affect breast feeding [4].

Table 1 Epidural versus non-epidural or no analgesia in labour (21 studies involving 6,664 women were included)

Outcome	Relative risk	95% CI
Oxytocin augmentation	1.18	1.03–1.34
Caesarean section	1.07	0.93–1.23
Instrumental delivery	1.38	1.24–1.53
Apgar score <7 at 5 min	0.70	0.44–1.10
Umbilical artery pH < 7.2 at delivery	0.80	0.66–0.96

In any case, the type of labour analgesia must be chosen by the woman together with her obstetrician and anaesthesiologist and should neither be forced nor refused.

References

1. Eltzchig HK, Liberman ES, Camann W (2003) Regional anesthesia and analgesia for labor and delivery. N Engl J Med 348:319–332
2. Sharma SK, Sidawi JE, Ramin SM et al (1997) Cesarean delivery: a randomized trial of epidural versus patient-controlled meperidine analgesia during labor. Anesthesiology 87:487–494
3. Task Force on Obstetrical Analgesia (1993) A report by the American Society of Anesthesiologists. Practical Guidelines for Obstetrical Anesthesia
4. Anim-Somuah M, Smyth R, Howell CJ (2005) Epidural versus non-epidural or no analgesia in labour [review]. Cochrane Database Syst Rev issue 4, art no CD000331. DOI: 10.1002/14651858.CD000331.pub2

PART II
Fetal Pain

Chapter 4
Ultrasound and Fetal Stress: Study of the Fetal Blink-Startle Reflex Evoked by Acoustic Stimuli

C. Bocchi, F.M. Severi, L. Bruni, G. Filardi, A. Delia, C. Boni, A. Altomare, C.V. Bellieni and F. Petraglia

The development of ultrasound techniques opened a window on the prenatal world. Since the early 1990s, bidimensional ultrasonography has played an important role in the study of certain fetal behaviours in attempts to understand fetal well-being. Certain fetal attitudes can be likened to those subsequently seen in newborns [1]. Study of fetal circulation by Doppler ultrasonography in parts of the fetal body such as the middle cerebral arteries has also clearly shown that certain pathophysiological and pathological conditions cause a redistribution of normal fetal circulation, indicating a change in fetal status.

The introduction of three-dimensional and four-dimensional (i.e. three-dimensional in real time) ultrasonography has enabled a more detailed morphological evaluation of the fetus, improving not only the definition but also the perception of certain fetal attitudes, such as facial expressions, in response to specific stimuli [2].

The uterus is an optimal, stimulating and interactive environment for fetal growth. Touch, the first sense that develops in the fetus, is fundamental for communication and human experience. The uterus is a protected but not isolated environment, where the embryo moves from an early age. Myocardial movements can be detected at week 4. These are followed by head rotation and movements of the arms and legs. By week 10, the embryo can be observed bringing hands to head, opening and closing the mouth and swallowing. By week 14, the repertoire of movements is complete. Fetal movements may be spontaneous, reflecting individual needs of the fetus, or may be evoked, reflecting fetal sensitivity to its environment.

The word *habituation* is used to indicate decrease or cessation of an evoked response after repeated presentation of the same stimulus. It is based on the brain's capacity to process short-term and long-term information. Habituation to visual, acoustic, olfactory and taste stimuli has been extensively studied in newborns [3]. Habituation depends on the capacity of the central nervous system to learn to recognize a stimulus: once habituation has occurred, the stimulus is ignored. Normal habituation to stimuli is therefore considered by researchers to express neurological well-being as it is based on *learning* [4].

With regard to learning capacity, fetal memory was first recognized in 1925. Recent experiments show that newborns have functional memory, development of which evidently began in the prenatal period. Prenatal memory is presumably rudimentary, developing quantitatively and qualitatively as the baby matures [4].

G. Buonocore, C.V. Bellieni (eds), *Neonatal Pain. Suffering, Pain and Risk of Brain Damage in the Fetus and Newborn*, © Springer 2008

Hypotheses about fetal memory functions currently being studied include recognition and bonding with the mother, breast feeding and the acquisition of language.

We know that newborns remember tastes and odours perceived in the uterus and that these prenatal perceptions may influence future preferences of the baby. Recent studies have shown that the uterine environment has an acoustic background consisting of sounds between 50 and 60 dB, among which the mother's voice, which is also transmitted by the bones, stands out. The sounds heard during prenatal life are recognized by fetuses and may have a relaxing effect on the baby.

The structural and functional development of hearing is complete around week 23 and this is the first sense to become completely mature. The fetus responds first to low frequencies, then to higher frequencies as gestation proceeds. Newborns have been found to recognize music that the mother listened to during pregnancy, and to recognize sounds that became familiar after week 30 [5].

Habituation to acoustic and vibrational stimuli has been tested by applying a sound at 80–110 dB every 5 s (range 4–7 s). At an intensity of 109 dB fetal heart rate increases, whereas at 103 dB fetal movements increase. Habituation is inversely proportional to gestational age [6] and does not depend on whether the fetus was quiet or active before application of the stimulus [7].

In our study [8] we evaluated the fetal blink-startle reflex, a complex reflex that appears around weeks 24–25, becoming very evident at week 28. Its presence indicates integrity of the seventh and eighth cranial nerves, and it is evoked by external stimuli. Long-term habituation of this reflex involves the brainstem. Electromyography (EMG) studies in adults have shown that it is altered in schizophrenia and psychoses and by caffeine intake.

Inclusion criteria of the study were: normal singleton pregnancy at 30–34 weeks with mothers fasting for at least 2 h, newborn 5-min Apgar score greater than 8 and negative neurological examination. The 22 pregnant women studied had a mean gestational period of 32 weeks.

A vibrational-acoustic stimulus, produced by an Amplicord model 95S laryngophone, was applied repeatedly to the maternal abdomen before the beginning of the routine ultrasound examination scheduled at 30–34 weeks' gestation (Siemens Sonoline Elegra Millennium edition with 3-D module). The blink-startle reflex was evaluated in a quiet environment, doing a coronal scan of the fetal face at suitable magnification. The stimulus was applied every 10 s until there was no fetal response to two consecutive stimuli.

The fetuses required four stimuli to habituate (mean 4.54, range 1–9). Delivery was spontaneous in 17 cases and by caesarean section in five cases. The newborns were 9 boys and 13 girls, all of normal weight (mean 3375 g). Mean hospital stay was 3.6 days (range 2–6 days).

The data of the present study, in which the blink-startle reflex was tested in a population of normal fetuses, provides a useful reference for our population. It will make it possible to detect future changes in this reflex, which could be a useful sign of neurological damage in high-risk pregnancies.

References

1. Da Silva FC, de Sá RA, de Carvalho PR, Lopes LM (2007) Doppler and birth weight Z score: predictors for adverse neonatal outcome in severe fetal compromise. Cardiovasc Ultrasound 5:15
2. Pilu G, Segata M, Ghi T et al (2006) Diagnosis of midline anomalies of the fetal brain with the three-dimensional median view. Ultrasound Obstet Gynecol 27:522–529
3. Gonzalez-Gonzalez NL, Suarez MN, Perez-Piñero B et al (2006) Persistence of fetal memory into neonatal life. Acta Obstet Gynecol Scand 85:1160–1164
4. Hepper PG (1996) Fetal memory: does it exist? What does it do? Acta Pediatr 416:16–20
5. Johansson B, Wedenberg E, Westin B (1992) Fetal heart rate response to acoustic stimulation in relation to fetal development and hearing impairment. Acta Obstet Gynecol Scand 71:610–615
6. Van Heteren CF, Boekkooi PF, Schiphorst RH et al (2001) Fetal habituation to vibroacoustic stimulation in uncomplicated postterm pregnancies. Eur J Obstet Gynecol Reprod Biol 97:178–182
7. Sarinoglu C, Dell J, Mercer BM, Sibai BM (1996) Fetal startle response observed under ultrasonography: a good predictor of a reassuring biophysical profile. Obstet Gynecol 88:599–602
8. Bellieni CV, Severi F, Bocchi C et al (2005) Blink-startle reflex habituation in 30–34 week low-risk fetuses. J Perinat Med 33:33–37

Chapter 5
Prenatal Affective Exchanges and Their Subsequent Effects in Postnatal Life

C. Dolto

This paper is the result of 23 years of haptotherapeutic clinical work with men, women, and children in difficulties and of pre- and postnatal haptonomic accompaniment of pregnancies, normal as well as pathological ones. After training as a pediatrician and several years of psychoanalysis and extensive work with Françoise Dolto (including attending her seminars), I discovered haptonomy in 1979. I committed myself to this practice, which seemed to promise many new possibilities for therapeutic fields, especially in relation to the prevention of problems in parent–child relationships. What this practice has actually brought has far surpassed my hopes.

It was Frans Veldman, a Dutchman, who discovered and developed haptonomy. He defines it as the science of affectivity and psychological–tactile (haptic) contact. It takes its name from the Greek verb *hapto*, which means "I touch in order to cure, to put together." It is a phenomenological, empirical (from the Greek *emperia*, experience), and human science; it enables one to approach the human being in the reality of the meeting, in the "here and now", in his or her entirety, avoiding any dissociation or hierarchy between body, psyche, and affectivity. Haptonomy allows us to step out of the psyche/soma dichotomy in which we have been enclosed for centuries.

Haptonomy proposes a sophisticated theory of the human person and human development very different from that of psychoanalysis, but cognitive discovery of this theoretical corpus will never enable real understanding of its essence. In haptonomy, understanding passes through feeling and experience before moving on to naming and analyzing. Hard cognitive work is, however, absolutely necessary to acquire a complete grasp of this complex thought.

Haptonomy is very much inspired by phenomenology. It builds a "phenomenality," which means a corpus of observable, identifiable, and reproducible phenomena which characterize the human affective life.

Haptonomy's theoretical, multidisciplinary, neurophysiological, anatomoclinical, and psychological background enables it to embrace the perpetual relationship which binds body and mind. Haptonomic phenomenality opens the door to a multilayered world where each level is related to the others through the effects of affective confirming contact and of personal experience of tenderness. The feeling of being complete brought about by this contact is essential for human development. This approach demonstrates that there is not one single memory but several memories, more or less archaic, more or less consciously active, which take place in our whole corporeality and the entries to which are sensorial. Emotions, being experiences, play a critical role in a person's overall construction as well as in the construction of memories. The hapto-psychotherapeutic method leads us to think that the question of infantile amnesia should be reconsidered in the light of new discoveries. Very often children tell the story of their birth, or describe it, without even knowing what it is. But this is has nothing to do with the phenomena of recovered memories.

Contact

The skin is tremendously important. It is the first sensorial organ the child may use in utero (the skin receptors are functional as of the 7th week of gestation) and the first organ of communication and exchange. The sense of touch is the one sense that is always reciprocal. In order to avoid this reciprocity (which they regard as a pitfall), medicine and paramedical disciplines have advocated an objective touch, which unfortunately results in a distance between the person approaching and the one being approached. Haptonomic phenomenality shows that the objective touch, being stressful, distorts the exchange. It induces reactions which hinder the clinical exam and warp the diagnosis. We use a particular contact, which needs to be learned and which we call psychotactile affective–confirming contact. Furthermore, perceptions and sensations coming from the interior of the body of the child mean a great deal to the child.

Affective Confirmation

According to haptonomy, the subject, being an autonomous source of desire, searches as early as conception for security. For this, the subject discriminates, very precociously, between what is good and what is bad for him. The psychotactile affective–confirming contact provides affective confirmation. It is indispensable for the proper development of the subject, who can then unfold all the possibilities gathered in his significant constellation, of which phylogenetic and ontological data are basic elements. In order to express itself, these genetic data need representation experiences, meetings, in which the subject's experiencing of his own goodness, in a mutually experienced affective environment of security, plays a decisive part. These exchanges, made of emotions, belong to the field of epigenetic evolution right from prenatal life. We know how important the epigenetic influence can be: it explains cerebral plasticity, which lasts until the end of life and enables one to escape the tyranny of one's genes, which is comforting.

The German notion of *Lust*, poorly translated as "pleasure" in English, is key to understanding the development of a healthy being. The experience of pleasure, in an environment of affective security and reciprocity, enables the individual to mature, his intellect to blossom, and promotes psychic well-being. Because of the structural importance of pleasure (*Lust*), we will speak about sensuality, and not sensoriality, from the beginning of fetal life. "Sensuality" means here sensorial perceptions effected by a feeling of pleasure or displeasure, of security or insecurity. This already plays a big part in prenatal life. To explain all this, haptonomy elucidated concepts and a theory which are impossible to give in detail here. However, I am going to cite some critical milestones to help you understand the following clinical elements.

Tone

"Representation tone" is a vital, integral, physical concept which embraces muscular tone, tension in tendons, ligaments, and capsules, interstitial tissue turgor, arterial tension, lymph circulation tension, as well as "psychotone" – the tension and strength of psychic expression. Representation tone is usually perceived as a quality of presence other people can feel and to which they react. In daily life, we speak about a nice presence, an anxious presence, an insecure presence, or, by contrast, a peaceful, open, and reassuring presence. Everybody knows how babies are receptive to the quality of presence of the people around them. They perceive the representation tone of nearby adults in an unaware way, on an affective level, prerational and prelogical. Reciprocally, they answer this with an adapted representation tone. Perception of this tone is even more important during prenatal life. When the child is in the womb, it feels all variations, whether comfortable or uncomfortable, secure or insecure, enabling freedom of movement or forced immobility.

Prenatal Accompaniment

We receive the couples in individual sessions, if possible starting right at the beginning of pregnancy, but most people start only at the 4th or 5th month of pregnancy. If a situation of distress arises for the child, mother, or father at a later stage in the pregnancy, an experienced haptotherapist can intervene to propose a different kind of work adapted to the urgent situation. I quite often receive women who are at risk of a premature delivery.

   This kind of approach relies on the desire and involvement of both parents. If the father does not wish to experience the pregnancy in this way, it is impossible to do it. Otherwise we would risk hindering the relationships within the parent-child triad in a potentially negative way, not knowing when and how their affective bonds will be touched. If the father has disappeared for good, the mother will be asked to choose another person to accompany her. This person – usually a woman – will not be a substitute for the father, who is present in the child what-ever the situation, but will enable the child to avoid a dual relationship with the mother, which would be oppressive for both of them. The third person, whether parent or not, is the one who opens up the relationship and thus prevents mother-child fusion.

We meet the couples at least eight times before the birth, more if necessary. The prenatal work must absolutely be followed by postnatal sessions, which are carried out in a very specific way. The last session, a very important one, takes place when the child stands up and starts walking. This accompaniment to parenthood cannot be compared with birth preparation, even though it certainly leads up to this major event, which is totally modified, particularly with regard to pain, by the develop-ment of the affective mother/father/child relationship.

The Intimate and the Extimate in the Secrecy of the Mother's Womb

From the Mother's Point of View

The psychotactile affective–confirming contact activates the subcortical channels as well as the whole limbic system and has direct effects on hormonal secretions (endorphins, cortisol) and on the muscular tone of the striated muscles, through the regulation of the neuromuscular spindles. The tone in the smooth muscles is mod-ified in relation with striated muscles but through ways which are still unknown.

As soon as a woman has established affective contact with the child she is bearing in her womb, her muscle tone modifies, creating an important change in her per-ceptions of her own body. She feels relaxed, at ease, and the muscle tone of her uterus becomes much more supple, even though she may have a hard time on an emotional or physical level. Her breath changes, without her even knowing it; her joints become more flexible. The child perceives these changes and immediately reacts to them by a slight movement of the spine.

Thanks to the possibilities offered by the affective contact, a woman can rock her child from within, inviting it to move towards her heart or her pelvis, to one side or the other, by the modification of tone that she thus induces in her womb. (The uterus muscles and abdominal muscles are experienced collectively as a tender, wel-coming place for the child.) The child is moved in the direction in which she invites it. If it is awake it goes along with the movement. In this way the mother can invite one twin towards the top and the other one towards the bottom, enabling a specif-ic playtime with each of the children. The discovery of these possibilities is always a very joyful surprise for the mother. It is even more important for a depressive moth-er, or for an ambivalent mother who hesitated to keep her child, or for a mother who feels powerless to help a child who is in danger.

From the Father's Point of View

The father first alerts the child to his presence through his manner of accompanying the mother. We teach fathers different ways to bring comfort to the mother, through rocking and easing the arch of the back. This simple contact, if it is affective-confirming, modifies the mother's muscular tone. It brings to her, and thus to the child, relaxation and ease. If a tense and tired woman lays down, the child starts moving intensely, in a jerky and abrupt way, enjoying the relative ease in the uterus provided by this position. However, if the father applies a light and tender touch, the child stops moving and remains quiet under his hand, which reassures both mother and child. After 5–10 min of quiet rest under this soothing hand, it will start its games again with a calmer, softer motion.

Fathers also play a very important part for their children through their voice. Unlike the mother's voice, which always vibrates the womb – the child's home – in the same way, the sporadic voice of the father envelops the child from different points and enables it to consider space. As of the third month of pregnancy, children react to a voice which is directed at them. If they like it, they go nearer (unless the mother prevents them from doing so). As is well known, until the beginning of the third trimester of the pregnancy hearing is not functional, but the skin, which is very sensitive, catches vibrations. I have been told that ancient obstetricians saw the skin of the fetus as a big ear. We experience this every day.

From the Child's Point of View

Let me say first that children give motor answers. They come nearer, go away, or sway by moving their pelvis, by leaning or pushing on the uterus wall, in an infinite number of variations. Twins play together. But motivity is a very subtle language; moving is not answering, stamping one's feet is not swaying. It is important to understand rhythm, amplitude, and the direction of each movement within the complexity of interactions between anatomy and physiology. It is clinically so obvious that parents very quickly feel these subtleties. When everything is fine, the mother accompanies her child from within in each of its movements, without even noticing it, thanks to what we call prelogical, prerational affective awareness. But she can also immobilize her child if she is not feeling well, if she is afraid, or if she is having a conflict, consciously or not, with the person who is trying to approach her child.

We find out that, long before birth, children are paying attention to everything that surrounds them: messages coming from their mother through the highly subtle interactions which bond them, but also exterior sounds and atmospheres. They receive them through their mother's feelings but also directly. They seem to be alert to any kind of sign. If a gentle and light hand calls them and then withdraws, they look for it: a real "hide and seek" game starts as long as the child is available. If the hand comes quietly, children will come and nestle under it and stay there. All children imperceptibly sway to the mother's breath. If we invite them to magnify their movement and they are awake and available, they take control of the swaying: its amplitude, rhythm, length, and direction. They can choose a lateral or up-and-down swaying, or a whirling around their axis, this movement being always very slow. These are real dances we perceive very clearly under our hands, to the point that the parents and the accompanying person feel the child is now rocking them. As of the 4th month of pregnancy, children are able to choose one kind of swaying, to memorize it, and moreover, to propose it to their parents, provided that the mother is available. Some children like only one kind of swaying, others change and go from one to the other every 5–10 s. We communicate with them through slight changes of hand weight and pressure. They make themselves known, each in their own way, surprising their parents, who thus get to know them long before the birth meeting. These dances are not only joyful manifestations, in reaction to our invitation or on their own initiative, they are also valuable signs of their state. A child who is not well will neither sway nor invite his parents.

These children – mobile, playful, attentive to the world and sensitive to tenderness – are the ones you take care of in your neonatal services, when the prematurity drama abruptly rushes them into an incubator. There they desperately suffer while discovering their new, constricted condition. They are pinned to their little bed by gravity, deprived of their usual reassuring gestures (sucking their thumb, playing with their umbilical cord, placenta, or feet, masturbating, or swallowing amniotic liquid) because of their lack of motor coordination. They have lost their freedom and any kind of potential initiative; they are now submissive and become passive. Many of them escape into their own world and anesthetize their perceptions; they dissociate themselves, which later on will influence their way of living. I am often brought newborns, just come out of neonatal services, who are suffering from what I call the "Sleeping Beauty syndrome." They are passive, waiting to be animated, to be brought back to life. You really have to call upon them strongly, physically but also on the emotional and psychological levels, to help them get out of this survival state, which is not really life.

Interactions Within the Triad

We are obviously in an extremely subtle universe. It is a tiny theater where each one plays a part. But we should not be fooled: even when the child is very small, even when its big answers seem small to us, in the palm of the hand, in the interior feelings of the mother, all of this is extremely precise. The accompanying person needs meticulous training and a long maturation period in order to be totally confident with his or her action. Such a subtle approach in such a sensitive period requires constant ethical reflection and responsibility.

The Exchange Dynamics

Through the tender contacts provided by its parents, the child receives affective confirmation, thanks to which it develops a feeling of a basic security. Reciprocally, the child answering to its parents gives them affective confirmation and they become mutually established. This ternary dynamic, this circulation of affective confirmations between the members (this is also the case in multiple pregnancies), is essential.

When a mother cannot be with her child, the child does not express itself much, and even if it moves, it never really enters a dialogue or proposes anything. When the mother is in conflict with the father, she does not accompany the child in its answers, and we can feel that the child has difficulty going closer to its father. A certain kind of "viscosity" shows the child's difficulty in clearing its own way, almost in spite of its mother. Sometimes the child is totally immobilized without the mother knowing what she is doing. Our work is to help her become aware of this and understand why things are happening this way so that she can overcome this difficulty. Most of the time it is quite easy to find the path back towards maternal feelings. What makes things difficult is anxiety, fear, and uncertainty. Modern medicine often creates these feelings to the point that they can become pathogenic. As of the in-utero life, the child looks for contact with its mother, and its quality of perception is stunning. If the child is in a moment of "dance," as I like to call these swaying sequences, it stops as soon as the mother thinks of something else and is no longer connected with it. These maternal withdrawals may be for insignificant or dramatic reasons. We adapt our approach depending on their origin. Sometimes they end up in laughter, when the mother got lost in a funny thought about the child, which led her to lose contact with the here and now of the relationship. Sometimes they end up in tears.

When the pregnancy is developing fine, all this brings pleasure to the parents and their child; they mature and change together. Newborns who have been well accompanied are born with excellent axial tone; they can immediately support their head. They are at the same time very awake, peaceful and smiling. They are usually rather precocious. With them you have to review pediatric semiology. Actually, this suggests that the haptonomic child is not precocious, but rather that all other children are slowed down by their lack of security and of affective confirmation. When one feels secure, one can go quicker and further.

Tragedies

Such a vast and complex subject deserves a lengthy treatment. What I feel I can strongly affirm today is that, as of the life in utero, children can help their parents going through difficult moments. Are they already driven by a therapeutic urge? This is difficult to prove, but they concretely assert themselves in crucial moments in a singular manner. When women are ambivalent, self-derogatory, feel guilty for not being the ideal mother they had imagined, hurt by receiving news of a developmental or inherited disorder in the child or by mourning, very often the child is the one who comes to help them in a most effective way. It goes up to her heart, where it rocks quietly, while she is crying or saying very painful or violent things. Sometimes it goes up to her heart in the deepest moments of despair. That is the child's way of telling her that she is a good enough mother. Even if she considered having an abortion or if she does not feel capable of being a mother, the child shows her that here and now she is its mother and that it is doing fine. It is obviously a great help for the mother, who is thus surprisingly able to get over very painful hurdles.

I must admit that I am not always able to say what is really happening during this period where we are in what I like to call the "totally intertwined mother and child." Who signals whom? It is not always possible to know, but a good accompaniment should only help to enable the bond to be permeable between the two, and then these astonishing and undoubtedly effective affective exchanges will happen under our eyes. When a woman is not well, the presence of the father (or the third person) is essential, because the child reacts to his approach and this helps the mother to come back to her child. A bipolar situation would lead them to a dead end, a total incapacity to change, symptomatic of a bond frozen in pain and reinforced by the feeling of guilt. But the third person, contacting the child, enables it to assert itself and find its path towards its mother alone.

The suspicion of a handicap, for which you might have to wait weeks before getting a confirmation or an invalidation, leaves long-lasting traces. Some parents come to me because they want to contact their child who is going to suffer a medically required abortion because of a severe malformation. These sessions are always moving and, strangely enough, both sad and happy. Parents have the opportunity to hold the hand of their condemned child until the end. During its short in-utero life, it will have received the goodness of their affection. That is exactly how you accompany a sick child to the end of its life, too. We work then for the future of the parents, and brothers and sisters already here or to be born. Experience has taught us that mourning is easier thus, whereas a mourning not properly done would weigh on several generations.

When the karyotype is normal, the child still needs to be helped to face life. Traces of these moments of doubt may poison the life of a family for years. Parents then have to retie a bond of confidence with it. The affective exchanges give the child the courage to live. This is pretty obvious when the child has to go through a very medicalized birth and a period in neonatal services. Children with a good accompaniment fight for life but remain quiet. They have developed a strong tolerance for frustration. This happens very quickly. Sometimes, very late in the gestation, we contact for the first time children who have endured a lot of ultrasound scans, or even some fetal surgery. Usually when I apply my hands, even though the mother knows and trusts me, the child goes through a moment of panic and of abrupt agitation before slowly regaining peace. These children are intensely open to contact, as if their ordeals had given them, more than others, a taste for communication. Experience shows that just one meeting with the parents can be enough; if they were really perceptive, the qualitative change is so radical that the child comes into the world quiet and peaceful, like one who has been accompanied for a long time.

Inhibition and depression are inseparable and it is interesting to discover that they are already tied in prenatal life. Depression inhibits maternal feeling or a mother's capacity to express it. She tightens her womb around the child and thus inhibits the relational dynamics of the child. This has definite effects on the constantly, quickly evolving child. Anxiety and anguish have the same inhibiting effects. The child withdraws, loses its impulses, just as if it were trying to fade away, then suddenly moves very abruptly or stamps his feet. Even if the child's development is not, most of the time, modified to the point of being medically serious, postnatal work with children shows that there are some traces left on the personality. Direct and indirect traces coming from the experience of the mother before and during the birth strongly influence her behavior with the baby.

There is no doubt that early prenatal ordeals or problems in the weeks following the birth leave much deeper influences than we thought until now. During the first 9 months of life, what Françoise Dolto suggested to us has been confirmed: children (and their parents) experience anniversary syndromes related to difficult periods of the pregnancy. The anguish of the 8th or 9th month can be considered as an anniversary syndrome of the anguish experienced by the mother (and/or father) and hence the child around its birth. If a child or its parents go through an ordeal at 4 or 5 months into the pregnancy, we have to recommend that the parents be very attentive to their baby when it reaches 4 or 5 months after birth. Very often they experience some sort of dysfunction. Merely speaking with them about what happened for them and their parents at 4 or 5 months in the womb makes everything return to normal. This is extremely important for premature babies.

This knowledge should not upset parents and practitioners facing traumatic events and their inevitable effects. On the contrary, knowledge of these powerful affective interactions around pregnancy enables us to help a great deal by giving the chance to speak about old or current difficulties in an affective proximity with the child. By allowing each other – especially the child – their place along with the dignity of their story, there is an immediate therapeutic effect and they become free of a burden that would have been too heavy. Some children start psychotherapy work around 6 or 7 years old with a pathology that makes me immediately think about a birth story. If this happens to be the case, we just need to tell the story, making the child the hero of the story – his story, from which he came out victorious – which proves he has powers which he can rely on. We then see the child straightening up and entering his epic, being proud of it, no longer crushed by it. This should always be tried before giving up when a child or a teenager who had early prenatal or postnatal problems is in trouble.

Memories of prenatal pain or difficulties during the first separation, the birth and the delivery, arise throughout life each time there is an abrupt transition, a separation, each time it is necessary to get mobilized to play a part in the world. In these moments, the effects of early maternal depression, prenatal tragedies, or traumatic birth reappear, particularly during adolescence (but also at the menopause or when retiring). We notice that the child or the teenager experiences heavy inhibitions to act, to dare, which might put them in a conflictual position, because they live with a strong desire to express themselves. The child who is born in fear, in anxiety, who has spent months in an incubator, who tried to be born, but in vain, or, on the contrary, was been born asleep when he was not ready, bears traces of this trauma, such as forbidden dynamics, lack of confidence in himself, in life, in others, lack of courage and strength. We can work on all this in a much simpler way than we think. It is surprising to see the power and duration of the positive or negative impacts of these first deep affective imprints. People suffer into old age because of the bond they had with their mother as small children, or in good cases are supported and carried through the hardest ordeals by the mutual trust and the affective security they experienced in the most archaic part of their life. The first psychoaffective layer has an incredible value.

There would be fewer pathological cases if we accepted the fact that the accompaniment of children and parents during this very sensitive period should be sustained by much ethical and political consideration, always trying to respect the necessity of mutual affective security. The first months of life, from conception, echo all the way along the path they initiate and unquestionably orient, and affect society as a whole. It is always possible to help later, but prevention avoids much suffering. These statements call upon our individual and collective responsibility.

Further Readings

Busnel MC (ed) (1993) Ce que savent les bébés. Édition Jacques Grancher, Paris
Damasio AR (1995) L'erreur de Descartes. Odile Jacob, Paris
Decant-Paoli D (2002) L'haptonomie. Que sais-je? Presses Universitaires de France, Paris
Dolto F (1997) Le sentiment de soi. Gallimard, Paris
Dolto C (1998) Le sentiment de sécurité de base. In: de Tichey C (ed) Actes du colloque "Psychologie Clinique et prévention", Nancy. Editions et applications psychologiques, Paris
Dolto C (2002) Sécurité affective, émotions et développement de l'identité: l'haptonomie. In: Mellier D (ed) Vie émotionnelle et souffrance du bébé. Dunod, Paris
Edelman GM (1992) Biologie de la conscience. Odile Jacob, Paris
Hochmann J, Jeannerod M (1991) Esprit est-tu là? Odile Jacob, Paris
Prochiantz A (1994) La biologie dans le boudoir. Odile Jacob, Paris
Tassin JP (1991) Biologie et inconscient. In: Le cerveau dans tous ses états: entretiens avec Monique Sicard. Presses du CNRS, Paris
Veldman F (1989) L'haptonomie, science de l'affectivité. Presses Universitaires de France, Paris
Veldman F (1990) Prolégomènes à une neurophysiologie de la phénoménalité haptonomique. In: Présence haptonomique no. 2, Paris
Veldman F (1999) Haptonomie, science de l'affectivité. Presses Universitaires de France, Paris, 1999

Chapter 6
Pain in the Fetus

G. Noia, E. Cesari, M.S. Ligato, D. Visconti, M. Tintoni, I. Mappa, C. Greco, G.P. Fortunato and A. Caruso

Introduction

All the recent data about the physiology of the fetus and its active role into the womb allow us to consider the fetus as a biological protagonist in the intrauterine environment. This capacity can be detected during both the embryonic and the fetal period. The pre-implantation blastocyst is biologically autonomous, because it can provide nutriments for itself during the trip from the oviduct to the site of implantation [1] and has an active role in the choice of the implantation site [2].

The relationship between the mother and the fetus starts immediately through biochemical dialogue, which is fundamental to good implantation: β-HCG induces the production of progesterone by the mother, while many molecules, such as early pregnancy factor (EPF), cause immunological tolerance in the mother [3]. During the fetal period also the conceptus is a "protagonist", promoting cellular traffic with the mother and to initiating labour. For these reasons, in the field of prenatal medicine, we need to consider the fetus as a patient, and the old concept of fetal well-being must be transformed in the new science of fetal medicine, which includes both treatment and diagnosis.

In our centre the main approaches to fetal therapy are transplacental, invasive ultrasound-guided and (at present only in experimental animals) open fetal surgery. Many of these procedures require transgression of the fetal body (e.g. thoracentesis, paracentesis, cystocentesis, pyelocentesis, shunt placement and fetal tissue biopsy) so, in our opinion, the important question is: does the fetus feel pain?

Fetal Pain Indicators

The definition of pain proposed by the International Association for the Study of Pain ("an unpleasant sensory and emotional experience associated with actual or potential tissue damage, that is described in term of such damage") is not adapted to dealings with the newborn or the fetus, because it assumes recognition and verbal expression of experience. We therefore need to use "indicators"

G. Buonocore, C.V. Bellieni (eds), *Neonatal Pain. Suffering, Pain and Risk of Brain Damage in the Fetus and Newborn*, © Springer 2008

of fetal pain. From the literature we can distinguish different types of indicators:

– Anatomical
– Cytochemical
– Neurophysiological
– Hormonal/haemodynamic
– Behavioural

Anatomical Indicators

Peripheral cutaneous sensory receptors develop early in the fetus. They appear in the perioral cutaneous area at around 7–8 weeks of gestational age and later in the palmar regions (10–10.5 weeks), abdominal wall (15 weeks) and then all over the body (16 weeks). The peripheral sensory neuron synapses on a dorsal horn interneuron, which stimulates the ventral horn motor neuron. These synapses are responsible for motor reflexes, which allow withdrawal of the limb from noxious stimuli (8 weeks) [4].

Many studies have focused on presence of thalamic fibre synapses to cortical plate to assess whether fetuses feel pain: there are no studies of thalamocortical fibres in relation to fetal pain, so we will analyse studies on other thalamocortical circuits. Kostovic and Rakic have shown that the density of cortical plate synapses increases around 26 weeks of gestational age, but histological analysis of eight fetuses showed that thalamic projection reached the visual cortex at 23–27 weeks of gestational age [5]. Krmpotic-Nemanic et al. showed that the auditory cortex was reached at between 26 and 28 weeks of gestation, and in one case cortical plate penetration was shown at 24 weeks [6]. These data are confirmed by a study of eight fetuses that demonstrated mediodorsal afferents to frontal cortex at 24 weeks [7].

Several studies have shown that before thalamic fibres reach the cortex they synapse on subplate neurons, that is a waiting "compartment" before the cortical plate. Thalamic projections reach the somatosensory subplate at 18 weeks [8]. There is evidence that neurons in the subplate zone initiate excitatory neurotransmission in the cortex, influencing the development of fetal cortical circuits [9]. These neurons may play a role in nociception transmission to the cortex.

Cytochemical Indicators

In the human fetus substance P appears in the dorsal horn at 8–10 weeks' gestation [10] and enkephalin at 12–14 weeks [11].

Neurophysiological Indicators

EEG is a measure of the electrical activity of cortical neurons. A primitive EEG is present from 19 weeks; from 22 weeks it is possible to recognize a continuous EEG pattern that is typical of the awake state and of REM sleep in the neonate. Somatosensory evoked potentials, which test the activity of the spinal cord, transmitting visceral pain sensation, are measurable from 24 weeks [12, 13].

Positron emission tomography has showed that glucose utilization is maximal in the sensory areas of the fetal cortex, implying high levels of activity [14].

In neurobehavioural studies in drug-addicted patients, the recording of fetal cardiotocographic patterns showed a cerebral involvement (between 27 and 35 weeks of gestation) of these patterns, demonstrating the presence of opiate receptors in these fetuses [15, 16].

Hormonal/Haemodynamic Indicators

Stress hormones, normally released by adults experiencing pain, are released in massive amounts by the fetuses subjected to needle puncture to draw a blood sample [17, 18]. Redistribution of blood flow occurs after acute painful stimuli [19].

In a fundamental study for research into fetal pain, Fisk has shown that after intrahepatic vein (IHV) procedures, fetal plasma cortisol and endorphin increased two to six times, whereas the fetal middle cerebral artery (MCA) pulsatility index (PI) decreased by two standard deviations, consistent with the centralization or "brain sparing" response. These hormonal and haemodynamic responses can be prevented by the administration of opioid analgesic (fentanyl) in the fetus [20, 21]. In another study, Fisk et al. demonstrated that noradrenaline (norepinephrine) and corticotropin-releasing hormone (CRH) concentrations increase after acute stress and that these events are independent from maternal responses [17, 22, 23].

The presence of opiate receptors in the fetal bladder was demonstrated by Noia et al., who measured the term of fetal micturition in drug-addicted patients by serial ultrasound evaluation until 18th week [16, 24].

Behavioural Indicators

Behavioural indicators of pain include withdrawing from painful stimuli, changes in vital signs, and facial movements. Preterm neonates of 26 weeks' gestation exhibit cutaneous withdrawal reflex after acute stress [25], and scalp sampling increases heart rate in some fetuses [26]. Some studies have identified a special set of facial expressions, similar to those of adult pain perception, that is present during invasive procedures in the premature neonate of 30 weeks' gestation [27–30].

Long-Term *Sequelae*

There is increasing evidence that early painful or stressful events can sensitize an individual to later pain or stress. Many invasive procedures resulting in acute pain, chronic pain, and prolonged stress – and also antenatal maternal psychological problems such as complications of past pregnancies or the current one, anxiety before and after invasive karyotyping, or mental disorders of the mother – can be dangerous if they happen during a critical window associated with epochal brain development.

Characteristics of the immature pain system in fetuses (such as a low pain threshold, prolonged periods of windup, overlapping receptive fields, immature descending inhibition) predispose them to greater clinical and behavioural sequelae from inadequately treated pain than older age groups [31]. Repetitive pain in neonatal rat pups can lead to an altered development of the pain system associated with decreased pain thresholds during development [32]. Evidence for developmental plasticity in the neonatal brain suggests that repetitive painful experiences during this period may alter neuronal and synaptic organization [19]. It is evident from animal study that prenatal stress can modify adaptive capacities throughout the entire life of animals: the hypothalamic–pituitary–adrenal (HPA) axis mediates the animal's responses to perinatal stressful events and thus serves as a neurobiological substrate of the behavioural consequences of these early events.

In an elegant study, Vallee et al. [33] showed that stress potentiates the age-related increase in circulating glucocorticoids levels in rats. They also demonstrated a reduction of hippocampal glucocorticoid receptors, which could be responsible, at least in part, for this prolonged corticosterone secretion observed after stress in prenatally stressed rats. In addition, they showed that prenatal stress enhances age-related memory impairments; thus, they hypothesized that elevated glucocorticoid levels could cause neuronal loss in the hippocampus, with subsequent impairment of cognition and memory [33].

In the primate model, exposure to a 2-week period of exogenous ACTH is associated with impaired motor coordination and muscle tonicity, reduced attention span and greater irritability [34]. Exposure to stress in utero is associated with higher levels of ACTH and cortisol in stressed newborns and with lower scores for attention and neuromotor maturity after birth [35, 36].

As we know, the HPA and immune systems are mutually regulatory and their interactions partially determine the effects of stress on immune function. Premature alteration of the HPA axis can cause alteration of the immune function, and thus prenatal stress could also have long-term implications in respect of infectious and autoimmune diseases.

In primates prenatal stress effects also appear to vary with the stage of pregnancy at which disruption occurs. Disruption during early pregnancy increases cellular immune responses, whereas prenatal stress exposure during mid- to late pregnancy can be immunosuppressive in adult offspring [37].

In rats, Gorczynski observed that stress-related immunosuppression (as measured by antibody responses and skin graft rejection) was most pronounced in offspring born from prenatally stressed dams [38]; prenatal stress accelerates the onset and increases the prevalence of diabetes in the non-obese diabetic (NOD) mouse model of insulin-dependent diabetes [39].

In humans, several studies demonstrated that early pain or stress (both in utero and in the neonatal period) impairs the physiological development of the nervous system, the HPA axis, and the immune system, producing long-term altered susceptibility to pain, to inflammatory diseases and to psychiatric disorders in later life.

It is important to understand the concept of "development plasticity", which means that one genotype can become many phenotypes depending on different environmental conditions during development [40]. Preterm neonates who had experienced 4 weeks of neonatal intensive care unit therapy manifested decreased behavioural responses and increased cardiovascular responses to the pain of a heel prick compared with neonates born at 32 weeks [41]. Taddio et al. demonstrated that children undergoing ritual circumcision immediately after birth without any kind of anaesthesia react more vigorously to vaccination at 2 months of age then those who received anaesthesia before surgery [42]. Other studies focused on hypersensitivity and hyperalgesia in the wound area after surgery [43].

The best evidence for an effect of maternal stress on the physical development of the baby comes from a study which has examined the links between prenatal stressors and fetal brain development. Information about stress was obtained from 3021 pregnant women by questionnaire. The 70 most stressed patients were compared with 50 controls. The authors found that antenatal stress is associated with a lower gestational age, lower birth weight, smaller head circumference and worse score on the neonatal neurological examination [44].

Zappitelli et al. showed that the mother's emotional state has a role in abnormal development of the neural dopaminergic system and can lead to attention deficit hyperactivity disorder (ADHD) in early childhood [45].

To test the role of maternal stress during pregnancy in psychiatric and behavioural disorders, a retrospective epidemiological study was conducted. One hundred and sixty-seven persons were identified whose fathers had died before they were born; a control group comprised 168 persons whose fathers had died during their 1st year of life. The number of diagnosed schizophrenics treated in psychiatric hospitals and the number of persons committing crimes were significantly higher in the index than in the control group. The results suggest that, especially during months 3–5 and 8–9 of pregnancy, maternal stress may increase the risk of psychiatric disorders in the children, perhaps mediated through the inborn temperament of the child [46].

The studies by Bracha et al. of schizophrenia in twins are very interesting. Concordances in subtypes of monozygotic twins can be used to investigate the influence of prenatal development in the aetiology of mental illness. The results of Bracha et al. indicate that simple monozygotic concordance rates may overestimate the heritability of schizophrenia, and that prenatal development may also be important in its aetiology. These authors thought that the second prenatal trimester is the critical period of the massive neural cell migration to the cortex and of the migration of fingertip dermal cells to form ridges. By determining differences in the fingertip ridge count of monozygotic twins discordant for schizophrenia, they demonstrated that prenatal stressors may contribute to the aetiology of schizophrenia. They analysed 30 pairs of monozygotic twins, 23 pairs in which the twins were discordant for schizophrenia and 7 pairs in which both twins were normal. In the discordant for schizophrenia pairs, no pair had the same number of digital ridges, despite their homozygosity. The authors concluded that twins, even homozygous ones, can react differently to the same maternal stress during the second trimester of pregnancy [47, 48].

It is our daily experience that invasive procedures can induce the pregnant mother to stop up "the channels" with her baby during the time when she is waiting for the answer on a prenatal diagnosis. Women who have an amniocentesis put their feelings on hold: what happens is a kind of separation of body and mind. The woman alienates herself from her own body and, by implication, from the child growing within her [49]. In our opinion this can be a severe insult to the developing fetus, and psychological support for these women could be an act of future social prevention.

Discussion

Some authors distinguish nociception from pain: the former is just an activation of anatomical pathway while the latter requires the presence of consciousness [50, 51]. Recently, Lee and colleagues published a systematic review that caused an interesting debate among scientists [52]. This is the first review about fetal pain. Many states in the USA are considering legislation requiring informed consent regarding analgesia for the fetus during abortion procedures after 20 weeks of gestation. Georgia and Arkansas have already approved such statutes [53, 54], so the authors ask: "Does the fetus have the functional capacity to feel pain?" They undertook a systematic review via PubMed of English-language articles on fetal pain. A multidisciplinary team revisited all the articles. They conclude that evidence regarding the fetus's feeling of pain is limited, and anyway it is unlikely that there is pain perception before the third trimester. The authors state that pain is an emotional and psychological experience that requires conscious recognition of a noxious stimulus. The presence of an anatomical pathway and other indicators does not mean that pain perception exists [52]. Derbyshire affirms that pain perception requires the development of representational memory, that is acquired only after birth [55]. Other authors state that studies on pain in preterm infants are not applicable to fetal pain perception, because "the fetus is actively maintained asleep (and unconscious) throughout gestation and cannot be woken by nociceptive stimuli". According to the authors, if the fetus is never awake it cannot be conscious and thus cannot feel pain. They try to demonstrated that the fetus is always asleep because in utero there are some chemical suppressors of fetal behaviour and cortical activity such as adenosine, allopregnanolone, pregnanolone and prostaglandin D_2. They also point to the warm temperature in the uterus and the presence of amniotic fluid, which induces sleep and protects the fetus from tactile stimulation. All these factors produce inhibition of cortical activity that is responsible, in their opinion, for the differences between fetus and neonate in their responses to stimuli, such as the response to hypoxia, which causes an arousal reaction in the neonate and depression in the fetus. In our opinion, it has been widely shown in the scientific literature that fetuses have access to a great deal of sensation in the uterus: they can perceive sound, the changing taste of the amniotic fluid, touch and pressure stimuli to the mother's abdomen, changes in light and dark and changes in balance [56–58].

The review by Lee and colleagues has many limitations. The first issue to discuss is the question of whether consciousness a condition necessary for the feeling of pain. According to the Oxford English Dictionary, pain is "a strongly unpleasant bodily sensation such as is produced by illness, injury or other harmful physical contact" [59]. Probably when a pregnant woman asks if her fetus can feel pain, she does not mean a conscious rationalization of pain. This is important for well-informed counselling of the women. Moreover, as Austin suggests [60], some of statements from which the author draws his conclusions must be questioned. The first is a semantic matter: according to the International Association for the Study of Pain, "each individual learns the application of the word [pain] through experiences related to injury in early life". This definition has limited biological and clinical application: in order to experience pain, the individual must first learn what pain is, and in order to learn what pain is, he must first experience it. This is a never-ending circular argument.

The second point is: Derbyshire claims that the perception of pain requires the development of representational memory; but, although memory may be necessary for the interpretation of pain, it is not for its perception. Even if the fetus does not recognize pain, the experience still remains unpleasant [60].

Despite their limited scientific significance, fetal pain indicators must be borne in mind especially because they are clinical signs of pain during surgery in unconscious and anaesthetized adults and paediatric patients [61].

The evidence that early exposure to noxious stimuli has adverse effects on future neural development is increasing [12, 62]. It follows that noxious stimulation may not need the presence of consciousness to alter the course of sensory development.

In our opinion this debate is strongly motivated by the question around voluntary termination. Claiming that abortion can cause fetal pain has important consequences for the personal ethics of both the parents and the clinicians – but this fear must not impede a scientific and honest search for the truth.

Conclusions

The American Academy of Pediatrics Fetus and Newborn Committee wrote a statement on the prevention and management of pain and stress in the neonate. The objectives of the statement are to:

– Increase awareness that neonates experience pain.
– Provide a physiological basis for neonatal pain and stress assessment and management by health care professionals.
– Make recommendations for reduced exposure of the neonate to noxious stimuli and to minimize associated adverse outcome.
– Recommend effective and safe interventions that relieve pain and stress [63].

Opioid analgesia for minor and major procedures has been shown in randomized trials to reduce metabolic and biophysical stress responses, postoperative morbidity and mortality and abnormal imprinting of subsequent pain responses in infancy [64].

Premature neonates are fetuses out of the intrauterine environment. Prevention or treatment of pain is a basic human right regardless of age and the humane care given to premature babies needs to be extended to the fetus.

We hope that all fetal medicine units will really take care of the well-being of the fetus, which is to take care of the well-being of the person for his entire life.

References

1. Buhi WC, Alvarez IM, Koumba AJ (2000) Secreted proteins of the oviduct. Cell Tissues Organs 166:165–179
2. Duc-Gorain P, Mignot TM, Bourgeois C, Ferre F (1999) Embryo-maternal interactions at the implantation site: a delicate equilibrium. Eur J Obstet Gynecol Reprod Biol 83:85–100
3. Di Trapani, Orozco C, Cock I, Clarke F (1997) A re-examination of the association of "early pregnancy factor" activity with fractions of heterogeneous molecular weight distribution in pregnancy sera. Early Pregnancy 3:312–322
4. Okado N, Kojima T (1984) Ontogeny of the central nervous system: neurogenesis, fibre connection, synaptogenesis and myelination in the spinal cord. In: Prechtl HFR (ed) Clinics in developmental medicine: continuity of neural functions from prenatal to postnatal life, vol 94. Lippincott, Philadelphia, pp 34–45
5. Kostovic I, Rakic P (1984) Development of prestriate visual projections in the monkey and human fetal cerebrum revealed by transient cholinesterase staining. J Neurosci 4:25–42
6. Krmpotic-Nemanic J, Kostovic I, Kelovic Z et al (1983) Development of the human fetal auditory cortex: growth of afferent fibres. Acta Anat (Basel) 116 :69–73
7. Kostovic I, Goldman-Rakic PS (1983) Transient cholinesterase staining in the mediodorsal nucleus of the thalamus and its connections in the developing human and monkey brain. J Comp Neurol 219:431–447
8. Kostovic I, Rakic P (1990) Developmental history of the transient subplate zone in the visual and somatosensory cortex of the macaque monkey and human brain. J Comp Neurol 297:441–470

9. Clancy B, Silva Filho M, Friedlander MJ (2001) Structure and projections of white matter neurons in the postnatal rat visual cortex J Comp Neurol 434:233–252
10. Charnay Y, Paulin C, Chayvialle JA, Dubois PM (1983) Distribution of substance P-like immunoreactivity in the spinal cord and dorsal root ganglia of the human foetus and infant. Neuroscience 10:41–55
11. Charnay Y, Paulin C, Dray F, Dubois PM (1984) Distribution of enkephalin in human fetus and infant spinal cord: an immunofluorescence study. J Comp Neurol 223: 415–423
12. Vanhatalo S, van Niuewenhuizen O (2000) Fetal pain? Brain Dev 22:145–150
13. Torres F, Anderson C (1985) The normal EEG of the human newborn. J Clin Neurophysiol 2:89–103
14. Chugani HT, Phelps ME (1986) Maturational changes in cerebral function in infants determined by 18FDG positron emission tomography. Science 231:840–843
15. Noia G, Arduini D, Rosati P et al (1985) Osservazioni preliminari sul behaviour fetale nelle gravidanze tossicodipendenti. In: Utopie e prospettive in ginecologia ed ostetricia. Monduzzi, Bologna, pp 349–357
16. Noia G, Caruso A, Mancuso S (1998) Le tecniche multiple invasive di diagnosi e terapie fetali e al storia naturale delle malformazioni. In: Le terapie fetali invasive, vol 4. Società Universo, Rome, pp 154–173
17. Giannakoulopoulos X, Sepulveda W, Kourtis P et al (1994) Fetal plasma cortisol and beta endorphin response to intrauterine needling. Lancet 344:77–81
18. Giannakoulopoulos X, Teixeira J, Fisk NM, Glover V (1999) Human fetal and maternal noradrenaline responses to invasive procedures. Pediatr Res 45:494–499
19. Smith RP, Gitau R, Glover V, Fisk NM (2000) Pain and stress in the human fetus. Eur J Obstet Gynecol Reprod Biol 92:161–165
20. Fisk NM, Gitau R, Teixeira JM et al (2001) Effect of direct fetal opioid analgesia on fetal hormonal and hemodynamic stress response to intrauterine needling. Anesthesiology 95:828–835
21. Texeira JM, Glover V, Fisk NM (1999) Acute cerebral redistribution in response to invasive procedures in the human fetus. Am J Obstet Gynecol 181:1018–1025
22. Gitau R, Fisk NM, Teixeira JM et al (2001) Fetal hypothalamic-pituitary-adrenal stress responses to invasive procedures are independent of maternal responses. J Clin Endocrinol Metab 86:104–109
23. Gitau R, Fisk NM, Glover V (2004) Human fetal and maternal corticotrophin releasing hormone responses to acute stress. Arch Dis Child Fetal Neonatal Ed 89:F29–F32
24. Noia G, Rosati P, Cicali B et al (1985) Urodinamica fetale: Studio ecografico preliminare in pazienti farmaco-dipendenti. Minerva Ginecologica, pp 681–684
25. Andrews K, Fitzgerald M (1994) The cutaneous withdrawal reflex in human neonates: sensitization, receptive fields, and the effects of contralateral stimulation. Pain 56:95–101
26. Spencer JA (1991) Predictive value of fetal heart rate acceleration at the time of fetal blood sampling in labour. J Perinat Med 19:207–215
27. Craig KD, Whitfield MF, Grunau RV et al (1993) Pain in the preterm neonate: behavioural and physiological indices. Pain 52:287–299
28. Xia C, Yang L, Zhang X (2002) Response to pain by different gestational age neonates J Huazhong Univ Sci Technolog Med Sci 22:84–86
29. Craig KD, Prkachin KM, Grunau RV (2001) Facial expression of pain . In: Turk DC, Melzack R (eds) Handbook of pain assessment, 2nd ed. Guilford Press, New York, pp 153–169
30. Craig KD, Hadjistavropoulos HD, Grunau RV, Whitfield MF (1994) A comparison of two measures of facial activity during pain in the newborn child. J Pediatr Psychol 19:305–318
31. Anand KJ, Phil D, Hickey PR (1987) Pain and its effects in the human neonate and fetus. N Engl J Med 317:1321–1329
32. Anand KJ, Barton BA, McIntosh N et al (1999) Analgesia and sedation in preterm neonates who require ventilatory support: results from the NOPAIN trial. Neonatal outcome and prolonged analgesia in neonates. Arch Pediatr Adolesc Med 153: 331–338

33. Vallee M, Maccari S, Dellu F et al (1999) Long-term effects of prenatal stress and post-natal handling on age-related glucocorticoid secretion and cognitive performance: a longitudinal study in the rat. Eur J Neurosci 11:2906–2916
34. Schneider ML, Coe CL, Lubach GR (1992) Endocrine activation mimics the adverse effects of prenatal stress on the neuromotor development of the infant primate. Dev Psychobiol 25:427–439
35. Clark AS, Wittner DJ, Abbott DH, Schneider ML (1994) Long-term effects of prenatal stress on HPA axis activity in juvenile rhesus monkeys. Dev Psychobiol 27:257–269
36. Schneider ML, Roughton EC, Koehler AJ, Lubach GR (1999) Growth and development following prenatal stress exposure in primates: an examination of ontogenetic vulnerability. Child Dev 70:263–274
37. Reves TM, Coe CL (1997) Prenatal manipulations reduce the proinflammatory response to a cytokine challenge in juvenile monkeys. Brain Res 769:29–35
38. Gorczynski RM (1992) Conditioned stress responses by pregnant and or lactating mice reduce immune responses of their offspring after weaning. Brain Behav Immun 6:87–95
39. Saravia-Fernandez F, Durant S, el Hasnaoui A et al (1996) Environmental and experimental procedures leading to variation in the incidence of diabetes in the nonobese diabetic (NOD) mouse. Autoimmunity 24:113–121
40. Barker DJ (1997) Fetal nutrition and cardiovascular disease in later life. Br Med Bull 53:96–108
41. Johnson CC, Stevens BJ (1996) Experience in a neonatal intensive care unit affects pain response. Pediatrics 98:925–930
42. Taddio A Kats J, Ilersich AL, Koren G (1997) Effects of neonatal circumcision on pain response during subsequent routine vaccination. Lancet 349:599–303
43. Andrews K, Fitzgerald M (2002) Wound sensitivity as a measure of analgesic effects following surgery in human neonates and infants. Pain 99:185–195
44. Lou HC, Hansen D, Nordentoft M et al (1994) Prenatal stressors of human life affect fetal brain development. Dev Med Child Neurol 36:826–832
45. Zappitelli M, Pinto T, Grizenko N (2001) Pre-, peri-, and postnatal trauma in subjects with attention-deficit hyperactivity disorder. Can J Psychol 46:542–548
46. Huttunen MO, Niskanen P (1978) Prenatal loss of father and psychiatric disorders. Arch Gen Psychiatry 35:429–431
47. Bracha HS, Torrey EF, Gottesman II et al (1992) Am J Psychol 149:1355–1361
48. Davis JO, Phelps JA, Bracha HS (1995) Prenatal development of monozygotic twins and concordance for schizophrenia. Schizophr Bull 21:357–366
49. Cederholm M, Sjödén PO, Axelsson O (2001) Psychological distress before and after prenatal invasive karyotyping. Act Obstet Gynecol Scand 80:539–545
50. Benatar D, Benatar M (2001) A pain in the fetus: toward ending confusion about fetal pain. Bioethics 15:57–76
51. Glover V, Fisk NM (1999) Fetal pain: implications for research and practice. Br J Obstet Gynaecol 106:881–886
52. Lee SJ, Ralston HJ, Drey EA et al (2005) Fetal pain: a systematic multidisciplinary review of the evidence. JAMA 294:947–954
53. Unborn Child Pain Awareness and Prevention Act (2005). To be codified at Ark Cde Ann 20–16–1101 to 1111
54. Woman's Right to Know Act. To be codified at Ga Code Ann 31–9A-4
55. Derbyshire SWS (2006) Can the fetus feel pain? BMJ 332:909–912
56. Lecanuet JP, Schaal B (1996) Fetal sensory competencies. Eur J Obstet Gynecol Reprod Biol 68:1–23
57. Kiuchi M, Nagata N, Ikeno S, Terakawa N (2000) The relationship between the response to external light stimulation and behavioral states in the human fetus: how it differs from vibroacoustic stimulation. Early Hum Dev 58:153–165
58. Visser GH, Mulder EJ (1993) The effect of vibro-acoustic stimulation on fetal behavioral state organization. Am J Ind Med 23:531–539
59. Concise Oxford Dictionary of Current English, 9th ed (1995) Oxford, Clarendon Press

60. Austin J (2006) The problem of pain. Rapid Responses to Derbyshire SWG Can fetus-es feel pain. BMJ 332:909–912
61. Sites BD (2006) Fetal pain. JAMA 295:160
62. Valman HB, Pearson JF (1980) What the fetus feels. Br Med J 26:233–234
63. Anonymous (2000) Prevention and management of pain and stress in the neonate. American Academy of Pediatrics. Committee on Fetus and Newborn. Committee on Drugs. Section on Anesthesiology. Section on Surgery. Canadian Paediatric Society. Fetus and Newborn Committee. Pediatrics 105:454–461
64. Anand KJ, Costun V, Thrivikraman KV et al (1999) Long term behavioural effects of repetitive pain in neonatal rat pups. Phys Behav 66:627–637

Chapter 7
New Insights into Prenatal Stress: Immediate and Long-Term Effects on the Fetus and Their Timing

K. O'Donnell and V. Glover

Introduction

A burgeoning literature emphasizes the importance of the in-utero environment on a range of fetal, neonatal, infant and adult health-related outcomes. This period of prenatal development, characterized by rapid growth and development, is a time of increased vulnerability, when intrauterine insults can have deleterious effects on emerging systems and structures. One important factor which affects the in-utero environment is maternal stress.

The immediate effects of prenatal stress relate to fetal well-being and the possible experience of the fetus. In this chapter we will discuss fetal stress responses, the potential for the fetus to feel pain, and the immediate and long-term effects of maternal stress on the fetus.

Fetal Stress Responses

Human fetal endocrine responses to stress have been demonstrated from 18 weeks' gestation. Our group first demonstrated increases in fetal plasma concentrations of cortisol and β-endorphin in response to needling of the intrahepatic vein (IHV) for intrauterine transfusion [1]. Fetuses receiving the same procedure of transfusion, but via the non-innervated placental cord insertion, failed to show these hormonal responses [2]. The fetal cortisol response, independent of the mother's, was observed from 20 weeks' gestation, but increased with gestational age. A similar but faster response is seen in fetal plasma noradrenaline (norepinephrine) levels to IHV needling. This, too, is observed in fetuses from at least 18 weeks, and is independent of the maternal response [3]. Human intrauterine needling studies that involve transgression of the fetal trunk have shown that brain sparing, as assessed by colour Doppler ultrasonography, affects the human fetus from at least 16 weeks' gestation, with a decrease in the pulsatility index of the middle cerebral artery, indicative of increased blood flow to the brain [4], and an increase in pulsatility index of the femoral artery [5].

Thus, from these studies one can conclude that the human blood flow redistribution response to an invasive stimulus is functional from at least 16 weeks' gestation, that the sympathetic system with the release of noradrenaline is functional from at least 18 weeks, and that the hypothalamic–pituitary–adrenal (HPA) axis is functionally mature enough to produce a β-endorphin response by 18 weeks and a cortisol response from 20 weeks' gestation.

Fetal Experience and Fetal Pain

Stress responses and blood flow redistribution do not show that the fetus is feeling pain. Production and release of stress hormones such as cortisol can be mediated by the hypothalamus, without involvement of the cortex or other higher brain regions involved in sentience. Although stress hormones are increased when an individual suffers pain, many other situations which are not painful, such as exercise, also increase levels.

We still do not know when the fetus starts to feel pain or when it starts to become conscious [6]. This subject is particularly difficult because the understanding of the physical basis of conscious awareness in the human adult is still limited. There may not be a single moment when consciousness, or the potential to experience pain, is turned on; it may come on gradually like a light on a dimmer switch [7]. Conscious experience is associated with the activation and inactivation of populations of neurons that are widely distributed in the thalamocortical system. The driving force of the activations of the thalamic cortical connections comes from lower in the brain stem, in the reticular activating system, which is located in the evolutionarily older part of the brain [8]. Waking consciousness is associated with low-level irregular activity in the electroencephalogram (EEG) ranging from 12 to 70 Hz [9]. However, sufficient conditions for consciousness are hard to establish. Edelman and colleagues have discussed evidence for consciousness in different animal species and concluded that birds may well be conscious, and it is even possible that the octopus is also [9, 10]. Both birds and octopuses have brains as different from an adult human as does a mid-trimester fetus, and their arguments suggest that we cannot be sure that for conscious experience it is necessary to have a functional cerebral cortex similar to that in the human adult.

For the fetus to feel pain there must be functional connections between the peripheral nociceptive receptors and the sites in the brain necessary for conscious experience of pain. There is considerable evidence, from positron emission tomographic studies in adults, that when pain is experienced as unpleasant, there is activation of a thalamic pathway which projects to areas of the cortex including the anterior insula, the anterior cingulate and the prefrontal cortex [11]. When these pathways are functional it is likely that the fetus or baby will feel pain. At earlier stages we have to make an informed guess.

The nervous system of the human fetus develops gradually throughout gestation, with the anatomical pathways and synapses forming first in the periphery and spinal cord and then moving upwards into the brain. In the brain the lower structures are connected first and then anatomical pathways are formed outwards towards the thalamus, the subplate zone (a region specific to the fetus which lies underneath the cortex) and finally the cerebral cortex.

The first essential requirement for nociception is the presence of sensory receptors, which start to develop in the perioral area at around 7 weeks' gestation [12]. Sensory receptors then develop in the rest of the face, and in the palmar surfaces of the hands and soles of the feet from 11 weeks. By 20 weeks, they are present throughout the skin and mucosal surfaces. In the first trimester stimulation of sensory receptors can result in local reflex movements involving the spinal cord but not the brain. Thus the fact that a fetus of 12 weeks will move away if touched is most unlikely to be associated with any conscious experience. As neurodevelopment continues these reflex pathways connect with the brain stem, and sensory stimulation can cause other responses such as increases in heart rate and blood pressure.

Assuming that activity in the cerebral cortex or subplate zone is necessary for consciousness, then for the fetus to be conscious of an external stimulus, these regions need to be connected with incoming nervous activity. Most incoming pathways, including nociceptive ones, are routed through the thalamus and start to penetrate the subplate zone from about 17 weeks. However, no human studies have examined the development of thalamocortical circuits specifically associated with pain perception.

Physiological evidence concerning the function of these pathways is even more limited than their anatomical development. There is evidence for a primitive EEG from 19–20 weeks. Sustained EEGs are obtainable from preterm infants of 23 weeks' gestation. Studies of evoked responses in preterm infants show that both visual and somatosensory potentials can be elicited from 24 weeks and are well developed by 27 weeks [13]. Clinical observations with preterm babies suggest that the nociceptive system is functional at 24–26 weeks [14], but when exactly it starts to function prior to this is not known.

Lee et al. [15] have stated that the capacity "for conscious perception of pain can arise only after thalamocortical pathways begin to function, which may occur in the third trimester around 29–30 weeks' gestational age". As discussed above, given the limitations of our current knowledge, this is unduly definite. Pain perception in the fetus may not use the same pathways as in the human adult, just as it may not in other species, such as the octopus [10]. Many fetal structures are different from those in the adult, and may function in a different way. We do not know that in the fetus thalamocortical pathways are essential for any perception of pain. Connections from the thalamus to the subplate zone may be sufficient, for example. If Lee et al.'s reasoning were correct, it would imply that the majority of premature babies in intensive care do not feel pain either.

We suggest that the current evidence, although still limited, makes it quite likely that the fetus can feel pain from 26 weeks, and very unlikely that it can feel pain before 17 weeks. It is possible that some sensory experience of pain may start by about 20 weeks.

Immediate Effects of Prenatal Maternal Experience on the Fetus

By mid-gestation a fetus is rapidly responsive to a diverse array of environmental stimuli [16]. Animal studies have demonstrated a myriad of negative effects upon the fetus, including changes in heart rate, blood pressure and reduced arterial oxygenation, providing evidence for direct effects of maternal stress reactivity on fetal physiology [17, 18]. More recent studies demonstrate that distinct fetal behaviours, such as changes in fetal heart rate in response to maternal psychological functioning, begin to emerge from 24 weeks [19].

Increases in fetal heart rate in the final trimester, following exposure to a cognitive stressor such as the Stroop test, were found to be greatest in mothers reporting increased depressive symptoms [20], and increased with gestational age. Paradoxically, this increase in the fetal response is in contrast to the progressive blunting of the maternal stress response to such stressors [21]. Both the maternal HPA axis and sympathetic system are found to become hyporesponsive to acute physical and psychological stressors toward the latter stages of pregnancy [21, 22]. But as gestation advances, and the fetus matures, an increased sensitivity to maternal input is observed.

Long-Term Effects of Prenatal Maternal Stress on the Fetus: Fetal Programming

The long-term effects of the fetal period have been highlighted by epidemiological studies carried out by Barker and colleagues [23, 24]. They have shown that poorer fetal growth is associated with increased mortality due to coronary heart disease, together with other aspects of the metabolic syndrome. A separate strand of research has examined the long-term effects of prenatal stress on neurodevelopmental outcomes [25, 26]. There is now good evidence that if the mother is stressed, anxious or depressed while pregnant, this increases the risk of her child having a range of behavioural, emotional or cognitive problems. The most consistently observed adverse outcome are symptoms of attention deficit hyperactivity disorder, which have been found in children between 4 and 15 years of age [27, 28]. However, other effects have also been described, such as increases in anxiety symptoms [27, 29] and externalizing problems [29]. Separate studies have shown an effect of prenatal stress on the cognitive development of the child, or its performance at school. These studies have focused primarily on infants and young children, although one study found an association between maternal antenatal stress and school marks at 6 years [30]. Huizink and colleagues [31] reported an association between maternal reports of daily hassles, pregnancy-related concerns and performance on the Mental Developmental Index (MDI) at 8 months of age. Bergman et al. [32] have also found that exposure to life events during pregnancy was associated with a significant reduction in the same scale in children of 14–19 months; there was no such link with postnatal life events scores.

Maternal exposure to traumatic events during pregnancy has also been associated with children's cognitive outcomes. Toddlers whose mothers were pregnant during the 1998 ice storm in Quebec – a disaster that resulted in the loss of electricity and water for up to 5 weeks – displayed lower MDI and language development scores compared to standardized norms [33]. Investigating cognitive development at later stages in childhood using assessments with greater predictive reliability remains an important next step.

It is also of interest that in one recent study of financially and emotionally stable women, there was a small but significant positive association between antenatal stress and both the MDI and physical developmental index (PDI) of the Bayley scales of infant development [34], suggesting beneficial effects of exposure to small to moderate levels of antenatal stress on child developmental outcomes.

Antenatal stress has also been associated with altered adult outcomes, although here studies have focused almost exclusively on psychopathology. Maternal exposure to traumatic events during pregnancy, for example, has been associated with increased lifetime risk of developing psychiatric disorders. In a retrospective cohort study, Van Os and Selten [35] demonstrated that the offspring of women who were pregnant during the German invasion of the Netherlands in 1940 were at significantly increased risk for developing schizophrenia. These results were replicated among a sample of Dutch adults whose mothers were pregnant during a devastating flood in 1953 [36]. An increased incidence of affective disorders has also been observed in individuals exposed in utero to the effects of the Dutch winter famine 1944–1945 [37, 38].

The studies described have reported associations between antenatal stress and a range of negative sequelae spanning infancy through to adulthood. However, other factors impinging on the development of emotional/behavioural problems must also be considered, ranging from shared genetic variance to indirect behavioural mechanisms of influence. The best evidence for an antenatal effect of psychological stress comes from those studies in which the association between prenatal stress and negative outcomes remains even after controlling for maternal postnatal anxiety or depression [27].

The periods of greatest vulnerability for fetal programming effects are not clear, and are likely to differ for different outcomes. For emotional and behavioural problems one study found greater effects with maternal anxiety at 32 weeks than at 18 weeks [27].

Underlying Mechanisms: HPA Axis and Associated Biological Processes

Investigators have focused primarily on the HPA axis in both mother and child as the primary biological mechanisms underlying the long-term effects of prenatal stress. In animal models, both rodent and non-human primate, the central role of the HPA axis in mediating prenatal stress effects in both mother and offspring is well established [39, 40]. Studies with non-human primates have provided convincing evidence that prenatal stress, and its associated increase in maternal HPA activity, is related to both short- and long-term negative sequelae in the offspring [41], including impairments in attention as well as heightened levels of anxiety. The central role of the maternal HPA axis has been demonstrated by showing that behavioural effects can be replicated by administering ACTH to the pregnant monkey [40] and abolished by adrenalectomy [42].

There is much less understanding of the mechanisms underlying the apparent effects of antenatal stress in humans, including the role of the HPA axis in mother or child. In one study, O'Connor et al. [43] found maternal antenatal anxiety at 32 weeks predicted children's morning cortisol concentrations after allowance was made for obstetric and sociodemographic factors. No links between children's cortisol and maternal anxiety or depression earlier in pregnancy or postnatally were observed [43].

There is evidence of a strong correlation between maternal plasma and fetal plasma cortisol levels [44], although fetal levels are about 10 times lower than maternal levels. Recent results demonstrate that the correlation between maternal and fetal cortisol only becomes significant by mid-gestation [45].

Based on the animal literature, a primary hypothesis would be that if the mother is stressed, her cortisol rises and this in turn crosses the placenta in sufficient concentrations to affect fetal development. However, problems remain with this proposed mechanism in humans. In particular, maternal cortisol responses to stress decrease markedly across gestation, such that by late pregnancy, the maternal HPA axis can be quite unresponsive [22, 46, 47]. Thus, at the time in pregnancy when there appears to be the strongest link between maternal and fetal cortisol, the maternal HPA axis becomes less sensitive to stress. It remains possible that at around mid-gestation, the maternal HPA axis is still responsive and there is passage of cortisol from mother to fetus.

However, other mediating mechanisms are also possible; they just have not been extensively studied in humans. For example, stress and anxiety cause substantial activation of the sympathetic–adrenal system and this could also be important. Noradrenaline does not appear to cross the placenta [3], but could have indirect effects upon the fetus by acting to cause contractions of the myometrium or by reducing uterine blood flow by affecting trophoblastic invasion. A second possibility, supported by recent in vitro and rodent work, may relate to the capacity of noradrenaline to downregulate placental 11βHSD-2, the enzyme which metabolizes cortisol [48].

Conclusions

It is suggested that extra vigilance or anxiety, readily distracted attention or a hyperresponsive HPA axis may have been adaptive in a stressful environment during evolution, but exists today at the cost of vulnerability to neurodevelopmental disorders. In animal models it has been demonstrated that effects of the in utero environment may be transmitted to the second generation. The effects of prenatal stress on child outcome should be a major public health concern.

References

1. Giannakoulopoulos X, Sepulveda W, Kourtis P et al (1994) Fetal plasma cortisol and beta-endorphin response to intrauterine needling. Lancet 344:77–81
2. Gitau R, Fisk NM, Teixeira JM et al (2001) Fetal hypothalamic-pituitary-adrenal stress responses to invasive procedures are independent of maternal responses. J Clin Endocrinol Metab 86:104–109
3. Giannakoulopoulos X, Teixeira J, Fisk N et al (1999) Human fetal and maternal noradrenaline responses to invasive procedures. Pediatr Res 45:494–499
4. Teixeira JM, Glover V, Fisk NM (1999) Acute cerebral redistribution in response to invasive procedures in the human fetus. Am J Obstet Gynecol 181:1018–1025
5. Smith RP, Glover V, Fisk NM (2003) Acute increase in femoral artery resistance in response to direct physical stimuli in the human fetus. BJOG 110:916–921
6. Glover V, Fisk N (1996) Do fetuses feel pain? We don't know; better to err on the safe side from mid-gestation. BMJ 313:796
7. Greenfield SA (1995) Journeys to the centres of the mind. Freeman, New York
8. Edelman DB, Tononi G (2000) A universe of conciousness. Basic Books, New York
9. Seth AK, Baars BJ, Edelman DB (2005) Criteria for consciousness in humans and other mammals. Conscious Cogn 14:119–139
10. Edelman DB, Baars BJ, Seth AK (2005) Identifying hallmarks of consciousness in non-mammalian species. Conscious Cogn 14:169–187
11. Lorenz J, Casey KL (2005) Imaging of acute versus pathological pain in humans. Eur J Pain 9:163–165
12. Fitzgerald M (1994) Neurobiology of fetal and neonatal pain. In: Wall P, Melzack ER (eds) Textbook of pain. Churchill Livingstone, Edinburgh
13. Klimach VJ, Cooke RW (1988) Maturation of the neonatal somatosensory evoked response in preterm infants. Dev Med Child Neurol 30:208–214
14. Fitzgerald M (1993) Development of pain pathways and mechanisms. In: Anand KIS, McGrath PJ (eds) Pain research and clinical management. Elsevier, New York
15. Lee SJ, Ralston HJP, Drey EA et al (2005) Fetal pain: a systematic multidisciplinary review of the evidence. JAMA 294:947–954
16. Austin MP, Leader LR, Reilly N (2005) Prenatal stress, the hypothalamic-pituitary-adrenal axis, and fetal and infant neurobehaviour. Early Hum Dev 81:917–926
17. Morishima HO, Pedersen H, Finster M (1978) The influence of maternal psychological stress on the fetus. Am J Obstet Gynecol 131:286–290
18. Myers RE (1975) Maternal psychological stress and fetal asphyxia: a study in the monkey. Am J Obstet Gynecol 122:47–59
19. DiPietro JA, Hilton SC, Hawkins M et al (2002) Maternal stress and affect influence fetal neurobehavioral development. Dev Psychol 38:659–668
20. Monk C, Sloan RP, Myers MM et al (2004) Fetal heart rate reactivity differs by women's psychiatric status: an early marker for developmental risk? J Am Acad Child Adolesc Psychiatry 43:283–290
21. DiPietro JA, Costigan KA, Gurewitsch ED (2005) Maternal psychophysiological change during the second half of gestation. Biol Psychol 69:23–38
22. Kammerer M, Adams D, Castelberg Bv, Glover V (2002) Pregnant women become insensitive to cold stress. BMC Pregnancy Childbirth 2:8
23. Barker DJ, Osmond C (1986) Infant mortality, childhood nutrition, and ischaemic heart disease in England and Wales. Lancet 1:1077–1081
24. Osmond C, Barker DJ, Winter PD et al (1993) Early growth and death from cardiovascular disease in women. BMJ 307:1519–1524
25. Van den Bergh BR, Mulder EJ, Mennes M et al (2005) Antenatal maternal anxiety and stress and the neurobehavioural development of the fetus and child: links and possible mechanisms. A review. Neurosci Biobehav Rev 29:237–258
26. Talge NM, Neal C, Glover V (2007) Antenatal maternal stress and long-term effects on child neurodevelopment: how and why? J Child Psychol Psychiatry 48:245–261

27. O'Connor TG, Heron J, Golding J et al (2002) Maternal antenatal anxiety and children's behavioural/emotional problems at 4 years. Report from the Avon Longitudinal Study of Parents and Children. Br J Psychiatry 180:502–508
28. van den Bergh BR, Mennes M, Stevens V et al (2006) ADHD deficit as measured in adolescent boys with a continuous performance task is related to antenatal maternal anxiety. Pediatr Res 59:78–82
29. Van den Bergh BR, Marcoen A (2004) High antenatal maternal anxiety is related to ADHD symptoms, externalizing problems, and anxiety in 8- and 9-year-olds. Child Dev 75:1085–1097
30. Niederhofer H, Reiter A (2004) Prenatal maternal stress, prenatal fetal movements and perinatal temperament factors influence behavior and school marks at the age of 6 years. Fetal Diagn Ther 19:160–162
31. Huizink AC, Robles de Medina PG, Mulder EJ et al (2003) Stress during pregnancy is associated with developmental outcome in infancy. J Child Psychol Psychiatry 44:810–818
32. Bergman K, Sarkar P, O'Connor TG et al (2007) Maternal stress during pregnancy predicts cognitive ability and fearfulness in infancy. J Am Acad Child Adolesc Psychiatry (in press)
33. Laplante DP, Barr RG, Brunet A et al (2004) Stress during pregnancy affects general intellectual and language functioning in human toddlers. Pediatr Res 56:400–410
34. DiPietro JA, Novak MF, Costigan KA et al (2006) Maternal psychological distress during pregnancy in relation to child development at age two. Child Dev 77:573–587
35. van Os J, Selten JP (1998) Prenatal exposure to maternal stress and subsequent schizophrenia. The May 1940 invasion of The Netherlands. Br J Psychiatry 172:324–326
36. Selten JP, van der Graaf Y, van Duursen R et al (1999) Psychotic illness after prenatal exposure to the 1953 Dutch Flood Disaster. Schizophr Res 35:243–245
37. Brown AS, Susser ES, Lin SP et al (1995) Increased risk of affective disorders in males after second trimester prenatal exposure to the Dutch hunger winter of 1944–45. Br J Psychiatry 166:601–606
38. Brown AS, van Os J, Driessens C et al (2000) Further evidence of relation between prenatal famine and major affective disorder. Am J Psychiatry 157:190–195
39. Weinstock M (1997) Does prenatal stress impair coping and regulation of hypothalamic-pituitary-adrenal axis? Neurosci Biobehav Rev 21:1–10
40. Schneider ML, Coe CL, Lubach GR (1992) Endocrine activation mimics the adverse effects of prenatal stress on the neuromotor development of the infant primate. Dev Psychobiol 25:427–439
41. Schneider ML, Moore CF, Kraemer GW et al (2002) The impact of prenatal stress, fetal alcohol exposure, or both on development: perspectives from a primate model. Psychoneuroendocrinology 27:285–298
42. Schneider ML (1999) Growth and development following prenatal stress exposure in primates: an examination of ontogenetic vulnerability. Child Dev 70:263
43. O'Connor TG, Ben-Shlomo Y, Heron J et al (2005) Prenatal anxiety predicts individual differences in cortisol in pre-adolescent children. Biol Psychiatry 58:211–217
44. Gitau R, Cameron A, Fisk NM et al (1998) Fetal exposure to maternal cortisol. Lancet 352:707–708
45. Sarkar P, Bergman K, Fisk NM et al (2007) Ontogeny of foetal exposure to maternal cortisol using midtrimester amniotic fluid as a biomarker. Clin Endocrinol (Oxf) 66:636–640
46. Schulte HM, Weisner D, Allolio B (1990) The corticotrophin releasing hormone test in late pregnancy: lack of adrenocorticotrophin and cortisol response. Clin Endocrinol (Oxf) 33:99–106
47. Sarkar P, Bergman K, Fisk NM et al (2006) Maternal anxiety at amniocentesis and plasma cortisol. Prenat Diagn 26:505–509
48. Mairesse J, Lesage J, Breton C et al (2007) Maternal stress alters endocrine function of the feto-placental unit in rats. Am J Physiol Endocrinol Metab 292:E1526–1533

PART III
Neonatal Pain

Chapter 8
Pain Assessment and Spectral Analysis of Neonatal Crying

C.V. Bellieni and G. Buonocore

Pain assessment in newborns is a widely debated topic. There are currently various methods of evaluating pain intensity in subjects who cannot express themselves in words, since pain can be assessed indirectly through the increase in plasma β-endorphin and catecholamines before and after pain, and through analysis of facial expression and complex movements of the extremities and of the changes in parameters such as oxygen saturation of the blood, heart rate and sweating of the palms. More than 30 neonatal pain scales exist, but almost none is actually used in clinical settings. Many of them are multifactorial, i.e. they simultaneously take account of fluctuations in oxygen saturation, blood pressure, and facial expression, but also score gestational age, behaviour and so on [1–9]. The more complex scales are good for research purposes, but only if we record the procedure in order to give the scorers the opportunity to assess the requested items in a later session. The most widely used are the PIPP (Premature Infant Pain Profile), NIPS (Neonatal Infant Pain Scale) and DAN (Douleur Aiguë du Nouveau-né) (see Chap. 9).

Most current scales are specific and sensitive but scarcely functional: caregivers are unable to take a blood sample or do some other painful operation and at the same time evaluate and time three or four physiological parameters, as required by certain scales. We recently published a work in which we studied the reliability of two of the most used pain scales for newborns [10]. We studied a group of babies who underwent a routine heel prick, and compared the scores for the babies' pain given by three different operators. Operator 1 was the nurse who was actually performing the heel prick; operator 2 was another nurse who did not perform the heel prick and was free to watch the baby and the saturometer closely; operator 3 was a third scorer who recorded the procedure through a video camera and scored the pain later. We studied two groups of babies, one made up of preterm babies, to whom scores were given using the PIPP, and another of term babies, for whom we used the NIPS. We used the score given by operator 3 as a reference score, because she could give the scores in a calm frame of mind and with the possibility of watching the video clip more than once. We found that, in both groups, both scorers 1 and 2 gave results different from those given by scorer 3; in the case of PIPP these differences were higher than in the case of NIPS. This difference may be due to the higher score range in PIPP, but could also be due to the greater complexity of the scale.

At all events, nobody can measure changes in heart rate, oxygen saturation, make the percentages of these variations or record to the split second the time babies spend frowning and simultaneously perform an invasive procedure. The need for an easy tool is clear.

Unifactorial assessment of acute pain through the observation of only one parameter (e.g. measuring crying length or heart rate variation) is unreliable, having low specificity and sensitivity. Post-surgery assessment of pain (assessment of chronic pain), by contrast, is easy and reliable using scales which are intended to evaluate the pain level every 4–6 h: the most used are the CRIES scale (C: crying; R: requires oxygen to maintain saturation greater than 95%; I: increased vital signs; E: expression; S: sleeplessness) and the EDIN scale (Echelle de la douleur et du inconfort du nouveau-né).

Can we find an easier and more reliable way to measure acute pain in newborns? Is crying analysis a possible path for this? Crying is simultaneously a sign, a symptom, and a signal, and is the infant's earliest form of communication [11], but the significance and meaning of neonatal crying are still unclear [12] because different crying features reflect not different causes (e.g. hunger, pain, fussing) [13], but the amount of distress caused [14–16]. Thus, gradations of crying may help a listener to narrow down the range of possible causes only with the help of contextual information [14, 16–19]. In the last few years, pain scales have been developed to discriminate levels of pain suffered by newborns [2, 5, 20–23], but in analyses of crying the level of pain that has provoked it is rarely considered [24]. Simple assessment of pain through measuring the duration of crying or other isolated parameters has been criticized for being neither sensitive, nor specific [25, 26]. In the 1960s crying was thought to be cause-specific (hunger, pain) [27], but recent reports have not found such a close correspondence, and this lack of specificity would prevent its use as a reliable pain indicator when crying is produced without contextual indications [28].

In 2003 our research group began analysing features of pain crying. We thoroughly assessed the characteristics of crying for different levels of pain: previous works had analysed pain crying, but without any regard to the different degrees of pain the baby was experiencing, with the single exception of one preliminary study [29]. We analysed a group of 56 healthy term babies during a common heel prick to obtain blood for routine analyses. We scored pain through a validated pain scale (DAN scale) and studied how the features of the crying varied according to the pain the babies were experiencing [30]. We studied three features: the pitch of the first cry emitted by the babies, the shape of the wave throughout the procedure, and, especially, the rhythmicity and constancy in time of the sound level. We chose these parameters because they are modulated by different parts of the nervous system. Cry pitch is due to vagus nerve tone, i.e. to the parasympathetic system: stress causes a decrease in tone, causing increased tension in the vocal cords innervated by the vagus nerve [31]. The rhythmic organization of infant crying is a complex phenomenon. Like other rhythmic patterns (sucking, walking), it has been correlated with central pattern generators [32], which are neural networks that produce rhythmic patterned outputs endogenously (i.e. without rhythmic sensory or central input). Last, the constancy of cry intensity is a sign of the persistence of the painful stimulus [17].

We saw that constancy of intensity increased with increasing pain. The basic frequency of the first cry did not increase until a certain pain threshold was reached (DAN > 8), after which the first burst was very acute. Rhythmic crying was absent up to a certain pain threshold (the same as for the above-mentioned basic frequency). We can therefore say that when pain passes a certain threshold, the characteristics of crying change: the crying becomes rhythmic and the first sound becomes acute, as if to express unbearable pain. We saw that, while crying constancy in time increases in accordance with the increase of pain, the other two parameters varied abruptly when pain exceeded a certain threshold. We supposed that this was a sort of protolanguage; it is unconscious, but finalized to express a state of extreme pain.

This was the premise of the development of the pain scale. We tried to verify whether these three items could be useful to score pain. We have already said that crying duration is not specific nor sensitive, but in this case we used not crying duration but some features of crying and integrated the three items to form a scale [33], of which we assessed the specificity, sensitivity, concurrent validity with another scale, interrater reliability and clinical utility. We called it the ABC scale (Table 1), because it used the "Acuteness" of the first cry, the "Burst rhythmicity" and the "Constancy" in time of the crying. J. Schollin in a recent issue of *Acta Pediatrica* [34] said that this scale was a good step in the field of pain assessment, because it was both easy and reliable. Examples of the different types of crying are available at the following URL: http://www.euraibi.com.

The last step in our research was validation of the ABC scale in premature babies [35]. In this case, too, we studied the specificity, sensitivity and reliability of the scale using statistical parameters. To make it easier to use the ABC scale, we developed software to measure pain automatically. This software uses the ABC scale and automatically analyses crying that arrives in the computer via a microphone. We have verified its validity and have published our data of our patented tool that we called "ABC analyser" [36]. It can be used to assess pain in nurseries and to train nurses who want to learn how to avoid pain in newborns.

Table 1 ABC scale for pain in newborns

Item		Score
Is the first cry acute?	No	0
	Yes	2
Are burst rhythmic?	No	0
	Yes	2
Is crying constant in time?	No (brief moan rather than crying)	0
	No (more than brief moan, but not constant)	1
	Yes	2

References

1. Franck LS, Greenberg CS, Stevens B (2000) Pain assessment in infants and children. Pediatr Clin North Am 47:487–512
2. Carbajal R, Paupe A, Hoenn E et al (1997) DAN: une échelle comportamentale d'évaluation de la douleur aiguë du nouveau-né. Arch Pediatr 4:623–628
3. Grunau RVE, Craig KD (1987) Pain expression in neonates: facial action and cry. Pain 28:395–410
4. Stevens B, Johnston C, Petryshen P, Taddio A (1996) Premature infant pain profile: development and initial validation. Clin J Pain 12:13–22
5. Krechel SW, Bildner J (1995) Cries: a new neonatal postoperative pain measurement score. Initial testing of validity and reliability. Pediatr Anaesth 5:53–61
6. Marceau J (2003) Pilot study of a pain assessment tool in the Neonatal Intensive Care Unit. J Paediatr Child Health 39:598–601
7. Peters JW, Koot HM, Grunau RE et al (2003) Neonatal facial coding system for assessing postoperative pain in infants: item reduction is valid and feasible. Clin J Pain 19:353–363
8. Guinsburg R, de Almeida MF, de Araujo Peres C et al (2003) Reliability of two behavioral tools to assess pain in preterm neonates. Sao Paulo Med J 121:72–76
9. Manworren RC, Hynan LS (2003) Clinical validation of FLACC: preverbal patient pain scale. Pediatr Nurs 29:140–146
10. Bellieni CV, Cordelli DM, Caliani C et al (2007) Inter-observer reliability of two pain scales for newborns. Early Hum Dev 83:549–552
11. Barr RG, Hopkins B, Green JA (2000) Crying as a sign, a symptom and a signal: evolving concepts of crying behavior. In: Barr RG, Hopkins B, Green JA (eds) Crying as a sign, a symptom and a signal. Cambridge University Press, Cambridge, pp 1–7
12. Choonara I (1999) Why do babies cry? BMJ 319:1381
13. Fuller BF (1991) Acoustic discrimination of three types of infant cries. Nurs Res 40:156–160
14. Gustafson GE, Wood RM, Green JA (2000) Can we hear the causes of infants' crying? In: Barr RG, Hopkins B, Green JA (eds) Crying as a sign, a symptom and a signal. Cambridge University Press, Cambridge, pp 8–22
15. Porter FL, Miller RH, Marshall RE (1986) Neonatal pain cries: effect of circumcision on acoustic features and perceived urgency. Child Dev 57:790–802
16. Wood RM, Gustafson GE (2001) Infant crying and adults' anticipated caregiving responses: acoustic and contextual influences. Child Dev 72:1287–1300
17. Corwin MJ, Lester BM, Golub HL (1996) The infant cry: what can it tell us? Curr Probl Pediatr 26:325–334
18. Zeskind PS, Marshall TR (1988) The relation between variations in pitch and maternal perceptions of infant crying. Child Dev 59:193–196
19. Lester BM, Boukydis CF, Garcia-Coll CT et al (1995) Developmental outcome as a function of the goodness of fit between the infant's cry characteristics and the mother's perception of her infant's cry. Pediatrics 95:516–521
20. Stevens B, Johnston CC, Petryshen P, Taddio A (1996) Premature infant pain profile: developmental and initial validation. Clin J Pain 12:13–22
21. Grunau RVE, Oberlander TF, Holsti L (1998) Bedside application of the neonatal facial coding system in pain assessment of premature neonates. Pain 76:277–286
22. Lawrence J, Alcock D, McGrath P et al (1993) The development of a tool to assess neonatal pain. Neonatal Netw 12:59–66
23. Sparshott M (1996) The development of a clinical distress scale for ventilated newborn infants: identification of pain based on validated behavioural scores. J Neonatal Nurs 2:5–11
24. Craig KD, Gilbert-Mac Leod CA, Lilley CM (2000) Crying as an indicator of pain in infants. In: Barr RG, Hopkins B, Green JA (eds) Crying as a sign, a symptom and a signal. Cambridge University Press, Cambridge, pp 23–40

25. Gallo AM (2003) The fifth vital sign: implementation of the Neonatal Infant Pain Scale. J Obstet Gynecol Neonatal Nurs 32:199–206
26. Gorski P (1984) Experiences following premature birth: stresses and opportunities for infants, parents and professionals. In: Call DJ, Galenson E, Tyson RL (eds) Frontiers of infant psychiatry. Basic Books, New York, pp 145–151
27. Wesz-Hockert W, Partanen T, Vuorenkoski V et al (1964) Effect of training on ability to identify preverbal vocalizations. Dev Med Child Neurol 6:393–396
28. Porter F (1989) Pain in the newborn. Clin Perinatol 16:549–1993
29. Johnston CC, Strada ME (1986) Acute pain response in infants: a multidimensional description. Pain 24:373–382
30. Bellieni CV, Sisto R, Cordelli DM, Buonocore G (2004) Cry features reflect pain intensity in term newborns: an alarm threshold. Pediatr Res 55:142–146
31. Zeskind PS, Parker-Price S, Barr RG (1993) Rhythmic organization of the sound of infant crying. Dev Psychobiol 26:321–333
32. Hooper SL (2000) Central pattern generators. Curr Biol 10:R176
33. Bellieni CV, Bagnoli F, Sisto R et al (2005) Development and validation of the ABC pain scale for healthy full-term babies. Acta Paediatr 94:1432–1436
34. Schollin J (2005) Can cry in the newborn be used as an assessment of pain? Acta Paediatr 94:1358–1360
35. Bellieni CV, Maffei M, Ancora G et al (2007) Is the ABC pain scale reliable for premature babies? Acta Pediatr (in press)
36. Sisto R, Bellieni CV, Perrone S, Buonocore G (2006) Neonatal pain analyzer: development and validation. Med Biol Eng Comput 44:841–845

Chapter 9
Analgesic Procedures in Newborns

L. Giuntini and G. Amato

> *"Pain is when you scream for help and no-one comes."*
> *(Elementary schoolchild)*

Fetal Period

Stress is already present in the fetal period and may be physical or psychological.

Physical Stress

Alcohol, smoking and drugs may cause behavioural disorganisation, up to temporary suppression of breathing in the case of maternal ingestion of alcohol. Ultrasound examination may also disorganise growth, as shown by studies of Newnham 1993 [1] and Evans 1996 [2]. According to the American Academy of Pediatrics, even noise may damage the fetus. Babies of mothers exposed to occupational noise during pregnancy showed statistically significant hearing deficit when they reached school age. It has also been shown that fetuses feel pain from week 18. This has given rise to the practice of using fetal anaesthesia for surgery or invasive diagnostic procedures in utero.

Psychological Stress

Psychological stress is as important as physical stress. Acute stress, such as grieving, can cause long-term psychological damage, and chronic stress has been shown to affect fetuses, being associated with premature birth, birth complications, or breast-feeding problems in babies whose mothers were unbalanced or had major psychoaffective disorders [3, 4]. All interruptions of affectivity during pregnancy with rejection by parents (e.g. awaiting diagnosis of pathological conditions) have repercussions on the fetus and its physiological parameters [5, 6].

Neonatal Period

After birth, stimuli vary, but if they are inadequate they can still affect development. Anand formulated a theory of hyperstimulation and hypostimulation [7].

Hyperstimulation

According to Anand and Carr, excessive neonatal stimulation leads to excitotoxic *N*-methyl-d-aspartate (NMDA) in many areas of the developing brain. The classic example is acute pain due to multiple invasive procedures, which may even cause intraventricular haemorrhage and leucomalacia due to intracranial pressure [7]. It has also been demonstrated that babies who were born prematurely, and were therefore subjected to many painful invasive procedures, have an anomalously low response to pain during infancy and greater somatisation in childhood [5]. The message is therefore that the clinical benefits of analgesia persist well beyond the duration of the therapeutic effect.

Hypostimulation

Prolonged separation of mother and newborn leads to anomalously exaggerated responses and alteration of neurotransmitter production [8]. The absence of stimuli increases apoptosis in the neonatal brain. If this is true, the clinical importance of preventing early insult and of developing appropriate analgesia and measures against neonatal stress (limitation of excitotoxicity and apoptosis) is evident. Pain experienced by babies has been underestimated throughout the world, not only in Italy. Before the above theories achieved scientific and clinical recognition, not only was neonatal pain ignored, it was even denied. It was thought that newborns did not feel pain and this idea was sustained with scientific arguments: (1) the immaturity of the neonatal central nervous system; (2) the difficulty doctors had in clinical recognition of pain; and (3) the assumption that the side effects of analgesia and anaesthesia outweighed their benefits.

In fact, the neuroexcitatory pain system controlled by NMDA (glutamate) and neuroquinine (neuropeptides) receptors develops in early fetal life, whereas the inhibitory system matures much more slowly and beyond birth. The inhibitory system consists of C fibres, descending nerve inhibitors, branches of which project onto the spinal cord only after birth, and neurotransmitters (GABA and glycine) that cause inhibition in adults but excitation in the immature nervous system. As a result, pain transmission through the spinal cord is amplified in newborns and the control system develops weeks later. On the other hand, opioid receptors are already active in fetal life. It can therefore be deduced that newborns feel pain more intensely than adults. The differences make babies even more vulnerable to nerve stimulation and, as we saw, continuous painful stimulation in a developing newborn has been demonstrated to modify its central nervous system [9, 10].

Pain Control

Pain control techniques should be used whenever possible before painful stimulation [11]. This is the basis of preventive analgesia. The aims are to:
– Minimise emotional problems
– Prevent CNS sensitisation
– Minimise release of pain mediators in tissues
– Decrease stress response
   Preventive analgesia also makes it possible to reduce the need for intrasurgical anaesthetic and also the demand for postoperative analgesia [12]. There are risks of various problems, psychological and physical, associated with not treating pain.
   Psychological problems:
– Fear and anxiety
– Behavioural and personality changes
– Vicious circle of chronic pain
   Physical problems:
– Increased mortality and morbidity after surgery
– Respiratory problems (hypoxaemia, reduction of coughing reflex, accumulation of secretions, infections)
– Cardiovascular problems (increased heart rate and blood pressure, vasoconstriction, increased oxygen consumption)
– Cerebral problems (increased intracerebral pressure, leading to risk of intraventricular haemorrhage and ischaemia)
– Skeletal muscle problems (muscle spasm, delayed mobilisation)
– Visceral problems (slowed gastrointestinal and urinary function)
– Delayed cicatrisation
– Stress response characterised by alteration of electrical signals and water balance (hyperglycaemia, osmotic diuresis)
– Immune depression

Multimodal Treatment

The multimodal treatment of pain combines pharmacological and non-pharmacological techniques in a safe, planned manner according to individual need. It therefore requires observation of the baby's physiological parameters and behaviour [13]. To do this, specific pain scores have been designed for newborns. In this age group, pain is evaluated through behavioural and physiological parameters, and in some cases stress hormone levels (Table 1). However, there are more neonatal pain scales according to the age of the patients, e.g. the Premature Infant Pain Profile (PIPP) for neonates aged 0–1 month (Table 2) [14], and the Objective Pain Scale (four-item OPS) for neonates aged between 1 month and 2 years (Table 3) [15]. During

Table 1 Behavioural and physiological parameters used for the evaluation of pain in newborns by a physician

Behavioural (observational)	Physiological	Psychological	
Position of the body	Reflexes	Projectional	Self report
Facial expression	Heart rate	Colours	Interview
Vocalisation pattern	Breathing frequency, Index fatigue	Forms	Questionnaires
Crying	Endorphin levels	Illustrations	Thermometer
		Drawings	Facial scales
		Visual analogue scales	

Table 2 Premature Infant Pain Profile (PIPP)

Indicator	Finding	Points
Gestational age	≤ 36 weeks	0
	32 weeks to 35 weeks 6 days	1
	28 weeks to 31 weeks 6 days	2
	< 28 weeks	3
Behavioural state	Active/awake, eyes open, facial movements	0
	Quiet/awake, eyes open, no facial movements	1
	Active/asleep, eyes closed, facial movements	2
	Quiet/asleep, eyes closed, no facial movements	3
Heart rate maximum	0–4 beats per minute increase	0
	5–14 beats per minute increase	1
	15–24 beats per minute increase	2
	≥ 25 beats per minute increase	3
Oxygen saturation minimum	0–2.4% decrease	0
	2.5–4.9% decrease	1
	5.0–7.4% decrease	2
	7.5% decrease or more	3
Brow bulge	None (≤ 9% of time)	0
	Minimum (10–39% of time)	1
	Moderate (40–69% of time)	2
	Maximum (≥ 70% of time)	3
Eye squeeze	None (≤ 9% of time)	0
	Minimum (10–39% of time)	1
	Moderate (40–69% of time)	2
	Maximum (≥ 70% of time)	3
Nasolabial furrow	None (≤ 9% of time)	0
	Minimum (10–39% of time)	1
	Moderate (40–69% of time)	2
	Maximum (≥ 70% of time)	3

the compilation of the PIPP, the important steps are to evaluate gestational age, score behaviour before potential pain (observe for 15 s), measure heart rate and basal oxygen saturation, and observe the baby and score the behaviour in the 30 seconds immediately after the painful event.

Table 3 Objective Pain Scale (OPS)

Indicator	Finding	Points
Blood pressure	+ 0% above preoperative BP	0
	10–20% above preoperative BP	1
	20% above preoperative BP	2
Crying	Absent	0
	Consolable	1
	Inconsolable	2
Movement	Absent	0
	Fidgety	1
	Thrashing	2
Agitation	Sleeping or calm	0
	Slight	1
	Intense, continuous	2

BP, blood pressure

Clinical Neonatal Pain Control

Pain control is possible with several methods, e.g. non-pharmacological techniques, topical analgesics, and systemic analgesia.

Analgesic Procedures in Newborns

Non-pharmacological Techniques

There are many non-pharmacological types of pain control, and they are of great significance for preventing suffering and reducing the use of analgesic agents. They include having a favourable environment, combining procedures, programming procedures on the basis of patient need rather than routine, avoiding heel-prick, decreasing noise and bright light, respect for the sleep-wake cycle, satisfying the sucking reflex, placing the baby in a comfortable natural position, changing its position from time to time (this includes ventilated babies), maintaining physical contact (stroking, rocking, massage), giving glucose solution (1 ml), and feeding or giving the dummy before painful procedures.

Topical Analgesia

A topical analgetic is EMLA (eutectic mixture of local anaesthetics), comprising lidocaine 2.5% and prilocaine 2.5%, total 5% (reduced risk of systemic toxicity after absorption). Application time is 1 h, the depth of action is 5 mm, and the duration of effect is 30–60 min. Melanin retards absorption. There is an associated risk of methaemo-globinaemia (reduced methaemoglobin reductase, fetal haemoglobin). Precautions to be taken in term and preterm newborns are to limit the contact surface and give no more than one application per day. Dosages: premature babies < 1500 g, 0.5 cm^2 (0.20 g); premature > 1500 g, 1 cm^2 (0.30 g); term, 2 cm^2 (0.50 g).

Regional Anaesthesia

Regional techniques, such as peripheral nerve blocks and central neuraxis blockade (spinal, epidural), are sometimes used to provide anaesthesia and analgesia for pro-cedures on the trunk or limbs, as an adjunct to general anaesthesia, and for postop-erative analgesia. Examples of regional nerve blocks include ilioinguinal and iliohy-pogastric nerve blocks, penile block, digital block, local infiltration, and intercostal nerve blocks. These techniques should be used carefully by health care professionals trained in their use and with appropriate and careful observation. In neonates, inter-mittent administration of dilute local anaesthetics with low-dose extradural opioids such as fentanyl offers less potential for the toxic effects of drugs than continuous infu-sion techniques with either drug alone. Accurate calculation is a particular concern in the care of preterm and term neonates, in whom differences in protein binding and metabolism can result in local anaesthetic drug accumulation and toxic effects [16].

Pharmacological Therapies

A knowledge of pharmacokinetics and pharmacodynamics in the neonatal period is necessary in order to use drugs. Major differences in this period involve distrib-ution volume, limited fat reserve, hepatic immaturity, renal immaturity with decreased glomerular filtration and reduced tubule resorption (lower metabolism and elimination), and qualitative and quantitative differences in plasma proteins. This means that the dose of most drugs must be reduced and the administration interval increased, at least in the 1st week of life. After the 1st month, the situation changes and there is an increase in metabolic capacity and distribution volume. Doses become equal to, if not higher, than those for adults.

Systemic Analgesia

Non-steroidal anti-inflammatory drugs (NSAIDs). Few papers have been pub-lished on the use of NSAIDs in newborns. Except for paracetamol, these drugs should not be used until renal function is mature. NSAIDs act by peripheral inhibition of eicosanoids, especially prostaglandins (responsible for pain associated with inflammation, together with histamine, serotonin and free thromboxane, in tissue lesions) [17]. They also decrease synthesis of oxygen free radicals, reducing migration of macrophages and inhibiting synthesis of NO. Unfortunately, they have a therapeutic threshold, their effect does not increase with increasing dose, and they must be associated with opioids (codeine, oxycodone).

Paracetamol. This analgesic is very safe and well tolerated. Unlike other NSAIDs, it does not have peripheral tissue anti-inflammatory properties but inhibits prostaglandins at hypothalamic level (pure analgesic and antipyretic). Its analgesic effect is directly proportional to its concentration in the blood. It is metabolised by the liver to active metabolites. Hepatic immaturity may be an advantage because production of toxic metabolites is believed to be lower. Because distribution volume is greater and elimination slower, it seems logical to give higher concentrations at longer intervals in this age group: 25–35 mg/kg every 6 h, maximum dose 60 mg/kg per day, instead of 15–20 mg/kg every 4 h. The injected form seems to potentiate spinal analgesia in the posterior body of the spinal cord (descending dorsolateral fascicle).

Opioids. Newborns are particularly vulnerable to side effects of opioids, such as respiratory depression. Other aspects to consider are higher rates of heart failure, the immature blood-brain barrier, the immature respiratory centre, longer metabolic times, a half-life up to four times longer, and wide variability between patients. This greater sensitivity of newborns does not mean that opioids should not be used, but it is important to select babies carefully, prescribe and prepare correctly, monitor side effects and monitor the infusion systems.

Morphine. This is the best known opioid in the neonatal period. It is rarely used, despite its low cost, because of its side effects, particularly in preterm babies. These are largely related to histamine release with bronchospasm and cardiocirculatory collapse due to vasodilation. Morphine causes less respiratory depression and thoracic rigidity than other opioids and may be used intravenously without respiratory assistance in the neonatal intensive care unit. A synthetic derived of morphine is fentanyl. Fentanyl has the following properties: it is a powerful analgesic, ten times stronger than morphine, fast acting (1 min) and with short duration (35–45 min); it maintains haemodynamic stability and is a poor sedative; it has a bradycardiac effect and induces thoracic rigidity; it is liposoluble, binds protein plasma and is metabolised in liver. Its half-life is up to 32 h in premature babies and infants. Guidelines for the administration of morphine and fentanyl are shown in Tables 4 and 5.

Table 4 Schedule for administration of morphine to neonates (with ventilation support)

	Intravenous bolus	Perfusion	Continuous infusion
Newborns < 34 weeks gestational age	5–10 g/kg every 10 min max. 20 µg/kg	3–40 µg/kg in 2 h	5 µg/kg per hour ↑ 2 µg/kg per hour every 4 h max. 15 µg/kg per hour
Term newborns	Max. 40 g/kg	50–100 µg/kg in 2 h	10 µg/kg per hour ↑ 5 µg/kg per hour every 4 h max. 20–25 µg/kg per hour

Without ventilation: 10–15 µg/kg per hour; ↑, may be increased by.

Table 5 Schedule for administration of fentanyl to neonates

	Intravenous bolus	Perfusion	Continuous infusion
Newborns < 32 weeks gestational age	0.5 g/kg every 10 min max. 1.5 µg/kg	3–40 µg/kg in 2 h	0.5 µg/kg per hour ↑ 0.5 µg/kg per hour every 4 h max. 2 µg/kg per hour
Term newborns	0.5 µg/kg every 10 min max. 4 µg/kg	1–3 µg/kg every 4-6 h	1 µg/kg per hour ↑ 0.5 µg/kg per hour every 2–4 h max. 2–4 µg/kg per hour

References

1. Jobe AM, Polk D, Ikegami H et al (1993) Lung responses to ultrasound-guided fetal treatments with corticosteroids in preterm lambs. J Appl Physiol 75:2099–2105
2. Evans MI, Hume RF, Johnson MP et al (1996) Integration of genetics and ultrasonography in prenatal diagnosis: just looking is not enough. Am J Obstet Gynecol 174:1925–1931
3. Relier JP (2001) Influence of maternal stress on fetal behavior and brain development. Biol Neonate 79:168–171
4. Richard S (1996) Influence du vécu emotionel de la femme enceinte sur le tempérament et la santé physique du nourisson. In: Relier JP (ed) Progrès en néonatologie, vol 16. Paris, Karger, pp 241–255
5. Monk E (2001) Stress and mood disorders during pregnancy: implications for child development. Psychiatr Q 72:347–457
6. Allister L, Lester BM, Carr S, Liv J (2001) The effect of maternal depression on fetal heart rate reponse to vibroacoustic stimulation. Dev Neuropsychol 20:639–651
7. Anand KJ, Carr DB (1989) The neuroanatomy, neurophysiology, and neurochemistry of pain, stress and analgesia in newborns and children. Pediatric Clin North Am 36:795–827
8. Kuhun CM, Pau KJ, Schamberg SM (1990) Endocrine response to mother-infant separation in developing rats. Dev Psychobiol 23:395–410
9. Fitzgerald M (1988) Hyperalgesia in premature infants. Lancet 1:292
10. Fitzgerald M (1989) Pain and analgesia in the newborn. Arch Dis Child 64:441
11. Bellieni CV, Buonocore G, Nenci A et al (2001) Sensorial saturation: an effective tool for heel prick in preterm infants. Biol Neonate 80:15–18

12. Chiaretti A, Pietrini D, Piastra M et al (2000) Safety and efficacy of remifentanil in cran-iosynostosis repair in childrn less than 1 year old. Pediatr Neurosurg 33:83–88
13. Wisman JS, Schecther NL (1991) Il trattamento del dolore nel paziente pediatrico. Pediatrics 4:112–119
14. Stevens B, Johnston C, Petryshen P et al (1996) Premature Infant Pain Profile: Development and initial validation. Clin J Pain 12:13–22
15. Nolent P, Nauquette MC, Carbajal R, Remolleau S (2006) Which sedation scale should be used in the pediatric intensive care unit? A comparative prospective study. Arch Pediatr 13:32–37
16. No authors listed (2000) Prevention and management of pain and stress in the neonate. Pediatrics 105:454–461
17. Berde CB (1989) Pediatric postoperative pain management. Pediatr Clin North Am 36:921–964

Chapter 10
Nonpharmacological Treatment of Neonatal Pain

R. Carbajal

Introduction

The alleviation of pain is a basic and human right regardless of age. It therefore seems unbelievable how long it took the medical community to realize that newborns are able to feel pain. During the last 15 years there has been a significant increase in our knowledge of pain in neonates, and broad areas of research have been addressed in the medical, nursing, psychological, neuroscientific, social, bioethical, and philosophical literature [1]. Despite these impressive gains, many of the previously identified and newer challenges remain, since we have not completely reversed the de-emphasis of infant pain [2], and no effective methods of preventing or treating pain for all infants in all clinical situations have been developed. However, the reason most of these challenges remain is because of the large gap that exists between published research results and routine clinical practice.

This article describes the nonpharmacological treatments currently available to alleviate procedural pain in neonates.

The Burden of Procedural Pain

Newborns routinely undergo painful invasive procedures, even after an uncomplicated birth. For obvious reasons, these invasive procedures that cause pain or distress are most frequently performed on infants admitted to the neonatal intensive care unit (NICU). For sick babies, multiple studies have documented a high frequency of invasive procedures during neonatal intensive care, particularly in preterm neonates, most of which are performed in the first week after birth [3, 4]. The most frequent procedures performed in NICUs are heel sticks, endotracheal suction, and intravenous line insertion [4, 5].

Despite increased awareness among clinicians about neonatal pain, management of procedural pain in neonates is not yet optimal, although recent surveys show that it is improving. In a multicenter prospective study carried out in France (The French Epippain study) on 430 neonates admitted to NICUs, 30 018 painful pro-

G. Buonocore, C.V. Bellieni (eds), *Neonatal Pain. Suffering, Pain and Risk of Brain Damage in the Fetus and Newborn,* © Springer 2008

cedures and 30 951 mainly stressful procedures were recorded during the first 14 days of admission. An analgesic treatment was given during 27.4% of painful procedures [5].

Analgesic Treatment

The goals of pain management in neonates are to minimize the pain experience and its physiological cost, and to maximize the newborn's capacity to cope with and recover from the painful experience while maintaining the best benefit/risk ratio for the treatment. Nonpharmacological techniques and pharmacological treatments are available for pain management in the neonate. Nonpharmacological interventions, which comprise environmental and behavioral interventions, have a wide applicability for neonatal pain management alone or in combinations with pharmacological treatments. These interventions are not necessarily substitutes or alternatives for pharmacological interventions, but rather are complementary [6]. Moreover, because painful procedures are extremely frequent in sick and preterm neonates, and because concerns exist regarding potential adverse effects of pharmacological agents, a growing interest has recently been developing in nonpharmacological interventions for procedural pain. These interventions can reduce pain in neonates indirectly, by reducing the total amount of noxious stimuli to which they are exposed, and directly, by blocking nociceptive transduction or transmission, or by activation of descending inhibitory pathways, or by activating attention and arousal systems that modulate pain [6].

Prevention

One of the most effective methods for reducing pain in neonates is to prevent it. Procedural pain can be minimized by efficient training of staff using indwelling lines for sampling, by planning procedures so that an analgesic approach can be considered [7], and by using mechanical devices if heel lance is necessary [8–10]. Compared to manual lancets, the use of mechanical lancets for heel pricks resulted in decreased behavioral and physiological distress and fewer repeated punctures [8, 9], increased volumes of blood, shortened time intervals for blood collection, and reduced hemolysis [11]. Heel warming, however, has not been found to have an effect on pain response [12]. It has also been shown that venepuncture is less painful than heel lance [13, 14]. A Cochrane review that evaluated venepuncture versus heel lance for blood sampling in term neonates concluded that venepuncture, when performed by a skilled phlebotomist, appears to be the method of choice for blood sampling in term neonates. For each three venepunctures instead of heel lance, the need for one additional skin puncture can be avoided [15]. Further well-designed randomized controlled trials need to be conducted, especially in preterm neonates, in whom venous access is technically difficult.

Another important prevention issue is to avoid systematic procedures; these must only be performed if they are absolutely necessary for the diagnostic and/or therapeutic management of neonates. In the French Epippain study, a 26 weeks' gestational age neonate underwent 95 heel sticks during the first 14 days after admission to the NICU (personal data). Given the burden that these procedures imposed on the neonate, one may ask if all these heel sticks were absolutely necessary.

Environmental Interventions

So-called environmental interventions aim to decrease the environmental stress of the NICU, where neonates are exposed to numerous repeated noxious stimuli including bright light, loud noise, frequent handling, and repeated painful procedures [6]. The reduction of lighting levels and alternating day and night conditions can reduce stress and promote increased sleep, weight gain, and the development of circadian rhythms [16, 17]. These findings suggest that physical environment has an effect (either direct or indirect) on the subsequent behavior of preterm infants and that exposure to night and day is beneficial. Another study has also shown a reduction of illness severity when light, noise, and handling were reduced [18].

Swaddling, "Facilitated Tucking", Positioning, and Touch

Swaddling is the wrapping of infants in cloth to restrict their movements. This intervention has been shown to reduce pain-elicited distress during and after heel stick in neonates [19]. This effect was, however, very modest. Fearon et al. studied the responses of 15 preterm neonates to swaddling after a heel stick [20]. They found that in neonates of 31 weeks' postconceptional age or older, the use of swaddling significantly reduced protracted behavioral disturbance.

Prasopkittikun and Tilokskulchai conducted a systematic analysis of studies carried out in Thailand on nonpharmacological methods of reducing pain responses to heel stick in neonates [21]. They found four studies that evaluated "hold and touch", "swaddling", and "positioning". "Hold and touch" consisted of cradling the baby in the mother's arms, while "positioning" consisted of using a blanket roll for containment, side-lying positioning with flexion of legs and arms. Pain measurement tools were not the same in all studies. The Neonatal Facial Coding system (NFCS) was used in two out of four studies. This score assesses only facial expression. The Premature Infant Pain Profile (PIPP) was used in the other two studies; it assesses facial expression, physiological (heart rate and oxygen saturation) changes, and contextual factors (gestational age and behavioral state). Regardless of which indicators were used, however, all study interventions were effective in attenuating neonates' pain scores [21]. Corff et al. found that preterm neonates who were arranged in a "facilitated tucking" (a side-lying or supine position with flexed arms and legs close to the trunk) demonstrated a significantly lower mean heart rate 6–10 min post-stick, shorter mean crying time, shorter mean sleep disruption time, and fewer sleep-state changes after heel stick than those who were the controls [22]. In a study carried out in preterm infants undergoing a heel stick, tactile and vocal stimulation were slightly helpful, but the use of a spring-loaded lance was most successful in reducing the distress [9].

Grunau et al. have studied the influence of position (prone or supine) on pain responses to heel lance in preterm infants at 32 weeks' gestational age [23]. Thirty-eight neonates were assigned to one of two positions during baseline and heel lance. The authors concluded that placement in the prone position is not a sufficient environmental comfort intervention for painful invasive procedures such as heel lance for blood sampling [23].

Nonnutritive Sucking

The pacifying effect of nonnutritive sucking (NNS) has been clearly shown in humans. Field and Goldson reported decreased crying with NNS in both term and preterm neonates during heel stick [24]. Shiao et al. reported in 1997 a meta-analysis of the effects of NNS on heart rate and peripheral oxygenation [25]. They identified four studies of the effect of NNS on heart rate without stimulations, three studies on heart rate during painful stimulations, and three studies on transcutaneous oxygen tension (tcPO$_2$). NNS significantly decreased heart rate without stimulations ($P = 0.002$) and during painful stimulations ($P = 0.0001$), and significantly increased tcPO$_2$ ($P = 0.0001$). As in all meta-analyses, the authors used the effect size as an index of how much difference exists between the groups. When effect size is based on means, it corresponds to the ratio of the difference between groups to the standard deviation. The total weighted effect size for heart rate without stimulations was small (0.17); however, it was large for heart rate during painful stimulations (1.05) and for tcPO$_2$ (0.69). Larger effects were noticed for preterm infants than for term infants and for longer NNS.

In infants of very low birth weight, Stevens et al. demonstrated that NNS is effective for relieving pain induced by routine heel lance procedures [26]. Corbo et al. investigated the effects of NNS during heel stick procedures in neonates of gestational ages ranging from 26 to 39 weeks [27]. NNS reduced the time of crying and the heart rate increase during the procedure but had no effect on respiratory rate or tcPO$_2$. In term neonates, other studies have also reported the analgesic effects of sucking a pacifier during heel stick [28, 29] and venepunctures [30]. Blass and Watt found that sucking an unflavored pacifier was analgesic only when suck rate exceeded 30 sucks/min [28]. Bellieni et al. have also shown in term neonates that NNS is

effective to reduce heel-stick-induced pain [29]. In their study, glucose plus sucking (elicited with the tip of a 1-ml syringe without needle placed in the baby's mouth)
was more effective than sucking alone.

Pinelli et al. reviewed in 2002 the available literature to look for negative effects
of NNS in high-risk full-term and preterm infants in neonatal nurseries [31]. From
this review, it appears that, although harmful effects have not been specifically studied, NNS in preterm and high-risk full-term infants does not seem to have any short-
term negative effects. No long-term data on the effects of NNS in high-risk full-
term and preterm infants are presently available.

Sweet Solutions

Sucrose

Blass and Hoffmeyer reported in 1991 the effectiveness of sucrose as an analgesic
agent for newborn infants during heel stick and circumcision [32]. Infants who drank
2 ml of a 12% sucrose solution (0.24 g) prior to blood collection cried 50% less
during the blood collection procedure than did control infants who had received 2 ml
of sterile water. Crying of infants who ingested sucrose returned to baseline levels
within 30–60 s after blood collection, whereas control infants required 2.5–3.0 min
to return to baseline. These findings provided the background for other studies that
confirmed the analgesic properties of oral sucrose.

Cochrane Review

A systematic review of the literature was carried out by the Cochrane
Collaboration in April 2004 in order to determine the efficacy, effect of dose, and
safety of sucrose for relieving procedural pain [33]. Twenty-one studies of a total
of 1616 infants fulfilled the selection criteria and were included in this review.
Of the 21 studies, 11 evaluated term infants, 9 evaluated preterm infants, and one
evaluated both preterm and term infants. The majority of infants (18 studies)
underwent heel lance as the painful procedure. In three studies, infants underwent
venepuncture. Sucrose in a wide variety of dosages was generally found to
decrease physiologic (heart rate) and behavioral pain indicators (mean percent time
crying, total cry duration, duration of first cry, and facial action) and composite
pain scores in neonates undergoing heel stick or venepuncture. Of the 15 studies
measuring heart rate/vagal tone, sucrose had a significant effect in reducing heart
rate in 8 studies. None of the 5 studies that assessed the effect of sucrose on oxygen saturation and respiratory rates reported significant differences between
sucrose and placebo groups. Different concentrations of sucrose administered at

varying time intervals have indicated that the greatest analgesic effect is realized when sucrose is administered approximately 2 min before the painful stimulus [33]. The authors of the review concluded that sucrose is safe and effective for reducing procedural pain from single painful events (heel lance, venepuncture). Regarding the optimal dose, the Cochrane review found that there was inconsistency in the dose of sucrose that was effective (dose range 0.012–0.12 g). In another meta-analysis carried out by Stevens on studies comprising primarily term neonates, doses of 0.24 g sucrose were most effective in reducing the proportion of time spent crying during 3 min after the painful stimulus [34]. A dose of 0.50 g provided no additional benefit.

Repeated Doses

Johnston et al. tested the efficacy of repeated doses versus a single dose of sucrose to decrease pain from routine heel sticks in 48 preterm neonates [35]. Infants in the first week of life with a mean gestational age of 31 weeks received 0.05 ml of 24% (0.012 g) sucrose solution or sterile water by mouth (a) 2 min prior to actual lancing of the heel; (b) just prior to lancing, and (c) 2 min after lancing. The single-dose group received sucrose for the first dose and water for the second and third dose; the repeated-dose group received sucrose three times, and the placebo group received only water. The pain scores (PIPP) group were obtained for five 30-s blocks from lancing. Both sucrose groups had lower PIPP scores (single sucrose pain scores: 6.8–8.2, $P = 0.07$; repeated sucrose pain scores: 5.3–6.2, $P < 0.01$) than water (pain scores: 7.9–9.1), and in the last block, the repeated dose had lower scores than the single dose (6.2 vs. 8.2, $P < 0.05$).

Doses, Age for Efficacy, and Recommendations

The studies reviewed above clearly indicate that sucrose reduces procedural pain from heel lance and venepuncture in neonates. Very small doses of 24% sucrose (0.01–0.02 g) were efficacious in reducing pain in infants of very low birth weight, while in term infants larger doses (0.24–0.50 g) reduced the proportion of time spent crying following a painful procedure [33]. These solutions should be administered approximately 2 min prior to the procedure. The analgesic effect lasts for about 5–7 min [36]. Therefore, if the procedure exceeds this duration, another oral administration should be performed.

Age parameters for efficacy are not very clear. Although sucrose continues to have an effect beyond the newborn period, some data show that this analgesic effect decreases with age and it is very modest at 2 months [37, 38]. A trial showed that 2 ml 24% sucrose was not effective in reducing pain in infants older than 30 days during bladder catheterization [39]. However, another study suggested that 2 ml 75% sucrose was effective in relieving crying after immunization in infants aged

2–6 months [40]. Similarly, Ramenghi et al. found that 50% sucrose resulted in shorter crying times, compared with 25% sucrose, glucose, or sterile water, for 4-month-old children [41]. They also found a trend toward shorter crying times for 2- and 3-month-old children receiving 50% sucrose, but it did not reach statistical significance. In spite of these conflicting data, an expert conference on pain reduction during immunizations recently considered that there seemed to be sufficient data to recommend sucrose use as a routine part of immunization administration for infants less than 6 months of age [42].

It has been shown that the responses to intraoral sucrose are neither specific to sucrose nor to the general class of carbohydrates, and that these effects are more appropriately understood as "sweetness" effects, since other sweet solutions are also effective [43]. The American and Canadian Pediatric Societies [44] as well as the Royal Australasian College of Physicians [45] have recommended the use of sucrose for such procedures as heel lances, injections, and intravenous line insertions.

Glucose

Oral glucose has also been shown to be effective in reducing procedural pain in neonates during minor procedures; 30% glucose has been effective both in term neonates during heel stick [46] and venepunctures [30], and in preterm neonates during subcutaneous injections [47]. Data on the comparison of the analgesic efficacy of sucrose and glucose are conflicting. In one study assessing pain with a behavioral pain score, the efficacies of 30% glucose and 30% sucrose were found to be similar [30]; in another study, changes in heart rate during heel sticks were similar among neonates receiving 33% and 50% glucose or sucrose [48]. However, in another study of 113 healthy term newborns, 30% sucrose was superior to 10% and 30% glucose solutions in reducing crying time [49]. In this study, neonates were randomized into four groups receiving 2 ml of 30% sucrose, 10% glucose, 30% glucose, or distilled water. Response to pain was assessed by mean crying time, recovery time, maximum heart rate, and percent change in heart rate at 1, 2, and 3 min. Mean crying times were 60, 102, 95, and 105 s in the sucrose, 10% glucose, 30% glucose, and placebo groups, respectively ($P = 0.02$). There were no differences among the groups in mean recovery time, maximum heart rate, and percent change in heart rate at 1, 2, and 3 min after heel prick [49].

Deshmukh and Udani studied the analgesic effect of different concentrations of oral glucose in preterm infants during venepuncture in a double-blind, randomized, controlled trial [50]. They randomized 60 infants to receive 2 ml of one of three solutions (sterile water, 10% glucose, and 25% glucose) in the mouth 2 min before venepuncture. There was a significant reduction in duration of first cry in the babies given 25% glucose compared with controls and those given 10% glucose. There was no significant effect on heart rate, respiratory rate, or oxygen saturation. There was no difference between 10% glucose and sterile water. Eriksson and Finnström studied whether repeated doses of orally administered glucose would cause tolerance [51]. They found in term neonates that the efficacy of oral glucose was not modified when 1 ml of 30% glucose was given three times a day for 3–5 days.

The coadministration of sucrose or glucose with a pacifier has been found to be synergistic [28, 30]. The association of a sweet solution and a pacifier provides a stronger analgesic effect than either one alone [30, 33].

Adverse Effects of Sweet Solutions

Six studies included in the Cochrane review [33] addressed the issue of adverse effects. One study [52] reported minor side effects in 6 out of 192 infants included in the study. One neonate who received water with pacifier choked when given the water but stabilized within 10 s. Three infants randomized to the sucrose group and two infants randomized to the water with pacifier group showed oxygen desaturation when the study intervention was administered. Each neonate recovered spontaneously with no medical intervention required [52]. In a study on the analgesic efficacy of glucose and pacifier in very preterm neonates during subcutaneous injections, slight (85–88%) and transient oxygen desaturations were observed in 7 out of 54 neonates during administration of interventions [47]. In five neonates it happened during administration of 30% glucose alone and in the other two during administration of 30% glucose plus the pacifier. None of the 24 placebo administrations elicited oxygen desaturations. For repeated administrations of sucrose in infants younger than 31 weeks' postconceptional age (PCA), Johnston et al. reported that higher numbers of doses of sucrose predicted lower scores for motor development and vigor, and for alertness and orientation at 36 weeks' PCA and lower motor development and vigor at 40 weeks' PCA [53]. These results need to be replicated because of their importance and also because the sample size was inadequate to show the same association in the placebo group, which could potentially be a methodological explanation for the observed results.

Multisensory Stimulation

Multisensory stimulation (massage, voice, eye contact, and perfume smelling) has been shown to be an effective analgesic technique that potentiates the analgesic effect of oral glucose during minor procedures [29]. This interesting method, also termed "sensory saturation", was developed by Bellieni et al. [29, 54]. This intervention consisted of: (1) laying the infant on its side with legs and arms flexed but free to move, (2) looking the infant in the face, close up, to attract its attention, and, simultaneously (3) massaging the infant's face and back, (4) speaking to the infant gently but firmly, and (5) letting the infant smell the fragrance of a baby perfume on the therapist's hands. A 33% glucose solution was also instilled on the infant's tongue with a syringe to stimulate sucking [29]. In a randomized study conducted on 120 term neonates these authors found that multisensory stimulation plus glucose was more effective in reducing pain from heel lance than glucose, sucking, or sucking plus glucose. They concluded that sensory saturation is an effective analgesic technique that potentiates the analgesic effect of oral glucose.

Skin-to-Skin Contact (Kangaroo Care)

Gray et al. found that 10–15 min skin-to-skin contact between mothers and their newborns reduces crying, grimacing, and heart rate during heel lance procedures in full-term newborns [55]. A total of 30 newborn infants were randomly assigned to either being held by their mothers in whole body, skin-to-skin contact or to no intervention (swaddled in crib) during a standard heel lance procedure. Crying was reduced by 82% and grimacing by 65% over the control group during the heel lance procedure. Heart rate also was reduced substantially by contact. Johnston et al. evaluated the efficacy of maternal skin-to-skin contact, or "kangaroo care," on diminishing the pain response of preterm neonates between 32 and 36 weeks' postmenstrual age to heel lancing [56]. They used a crossover design, in which infants served as their own controls. In the kangaroo care group, the neonate was held in skin-to-skin contact for 30 min before the heel stick and remained in contact for the duration of the procedure. In the control condition, the neonate was in the prone position in the incubator. The ordering of conditions was random. All procedures were videotaped. Research assistants who were naïve to the purpose of the study coded video recordings that were taken with the camera positioned on the neonate's face so that an observer could not tell whether the neonate was being held or was in the incubator. Heart rate and oxygen levels were continuously monitored by computer. Pain was assessed with the PIPP score from videotapes. PIPP scores across the first 90 s from the heel-lancing procedure were significantly lower by 2 points in the kangaroo care condition.

Given the analgesic effectiveness of skin-to-skin contact shown in the above studies, and the fact that parents of neonates in critical care units want to participate more in comforting their infants, kangaroo care is a potentially beneficial strategy for promoting family health. Nonetheless, further research is warranted before kangaroo care can be recommended as a standard practice for procedural pain control.

Breastfeeding Analgesia

Breastfeeding maintained throughout a procedure has been shown to be a potent analgesic to relieve procedural pain in term neonates [57–60]. In one study, neonates who were held and breastfed by their mothers during heel lance and blood collection had a reduction in crying of 91% and grimacing of 84%, as compared to infants who had the same blood test while being swaddled in their bassinets [57]. In another study, Carbajal et al. randomized 180 term newborns undergoing venepunctures to receive four different analgesic interventions [58]. Venepunctures were performed in the first group while neonates were breastfeeding and in the second group while neonates were held in their mothers' arms without breastfeeding. In the third group neonates received 1 ml of placebo (sterile water) 2 min prior to venipuncture, and in the fourth group neonates received 1 ml of 30% glucose 1 min prior to venipuncture and sucked a pacifier before and throughout the procedure. Pain-related behaviors during venepunctures were evaluated using two infant pain scales (DAN scale and PIPP scale). Significant reductions in DAN (Douleur Aiguë Nouveau-né) and PIPP scores were noted for the breastfeeding and glucose plus pacifier groups from the other two groups. Although DAN pain scores were lower in the breastfeeding group as compared to the glucose plus pacifier group, this difference did not reach statistical significance [58]. More recently, Phillips et al. compared the analgesic effect of breastfeeding and pacifier use with maternal holding in term infants undergoing blood collection via heel sticks in a randomized controlled study [60]. A total of 96 infants were randomized to three groups for analgesia: (1) breastfeeding, (2) pacifier use while held by mothers, (3) pacifier use while held by research assistants (nonmothers). The authors found that breastfeeding is more analgesic than pacifier use with nonmaternal holding. They also concluded that maternal holding with either breastfeeding or pacifier use is more analgesic than nonmaternal holding with pacifier use. Shendurnikar and Ghandi randomized 100 neonates so that half of them were heel lanced while being breastfed whereas the other half were heel lanced after being swaddled and kept in a cradle away from their mothers [59]. Statistically lower pain scores were observed at 1, 5, and 15 min after lancing in the breastfed group. Two other studies have evaluated the analgesic efficacy of breastfeeding prior to a painful procedure but discontinued during the procedure [61, 62]. These studies have shown that if breastfeeding is not maintained during the procedure, there is no analgesic effect.

Breast Milk

Studies on the analgesic effects of supplemental breast milk to reduce procedural pain in neonates have yielded conflicting results [46, 63–67]. In these studies 1–2 ml of breast milk, which contains 7% lactose, was placed in the infant's mouth via a syringe [46, 63–65, 67] or a special cup [66]. Term neonates were given 2 ml of breast milk, and in the only study that included preterm and term neonates [46], infants were given 1 ml of breast milk. Shah et al. have conducted a Cochrane review on these studies and concluded that neonates given supplemental breast milk had significantly less increase in heart rate and NFCS compared to placebo groups [68]. However, the difference in the duration of crying and oxygen saturation change between the supplemental breast milk group and the placebo group were not statistically significant. Overall, results were conflicting; for instance, Blass and colleagues [63] found that although colostrum delivered by syringe or on a pacifier did not reduce crying or grimacing relative to control infants who received water, it did prevent the increase in heart rate. Moreover, it was also found that supplemental breast milk did not compare favorably to concentrated glucose or sucrose, as reflected by higher increases in heart rate changes and duration of crying time in the breast milk group. Thus, the available evidence does not support the use of milk as the sole intervention to alleviate procedural pain.

Music

Music has been used since ancient times to enhance well-being and reduce pain and suffering [69]. Music is defined as an intentional auditory stimulus with organized elements including melody, rhythm, harmony, timbre, form, and style. By contrast, environmental sounds that exist without controls for volume or cause/effect relations are perceived as noise [69]. Music is ubiquitous in all human cultures and is listened to by persons of all ages, races, and ethnic backgrounds. Music and music therapy may benefit patients both directly and indirectly. Music has physiological, psychological, and socioemotional direct effects. It may also affect patients indirectly through its effects on caregivers' attitudes and behaviors [69].

Bo and Callaghan have tested the effect of NNS, music therapy (MT), and combined NNS and MT (NNS+MT), versus no intervention, on heart rate, $tcPO_2$ levels, and pain behavior of neonates in NICUs having blood taken by a heel-stick procedure [70]. The researchers used a within-subjects, repeated-measures, counterbalancing design. Each trial consisted of three periods of data collection: a baseline 1 min before the heel-stick procedure, each minute during 5 min of intervention, and each minute for 8 min after the heel stick. During the MT intervention the researcher played intrauterine maternal pulse sounds with soothing music through a cassette recorder placed near the neonate's head using the same volume each time. In the combined MT+NNS intervention, the neonates had the intrauterine sounds and a latex nipple. The authors found in 27 neonates of 30–41 weeks' gestational age that the three comfort interventions significantly reduced neonates' heart rate, improved their $tcPO_2$ levels, and reduced their pain behavior. NNS+MT had the strongest effect on neonates' $tcPO_2$ levels and pain behavior; MT alone had the strongest effect on neonates' heart rate. Butt and Kisilevsky examined the physiological and behavioral effects of music during recovery from heel lance in 14 preterm infants at 29–36 weeks' PCA in a crossover study [71]. Infants were tested on two occasions: during a music condition and during a no-music control condition. Each condition was videotaped during three periods: baseline, heel lance, and recovery. Heel lance elicited a stress response (i.e., increased heart rate, decreased oxygen saturation, increased state of arousal, and increased facial actions indicative of pain) in both age groups. The stress response was greater in infants of PCA greater than 31 weeks. During recovery, these infants had a more rapid return of heart rate, behavioral state, and facial expressions of pain to baseline levels in the presence of compared to the absence of music. The authors concluded that music is an effective intervention following a stress-provoking stimulus in infants older than 31 weeks PCA [71]. The limitations of this study include the small sample size and the absence of order effect testing (i.e., if the order of music and no-music conditions affected the outcome).

Although methodological limitations exist, results of published studies suggest that music may be useful in reducing procedural pain in neonates. If music is used, it should probably not be provided for longer than 15 min per intervention due to the risk of sensory overload [72].

Conclusions

As stated in the introduction, the alleviation of pain is a basic need and human right regardless of age. Thus, the prevention and treatment of neonatal pain is essential. Procedural pain is the principal source of pain in sick or preterm neonates. These neonates experience numerous heel sticks, tracheal aspirations, venous and arterial punctures, gastric tube placements, and tracheal intubations. Epidemiological studies still show the need to improve procedural pain management in neonates. Several nonpharmacological interventions are effective in reducing procedural pain in neonates. These interventions are simple, feasible, and accessible and can be easily given by those caring for neonates. Using these interventions may also be cost-effective because they involve minimal effort and time and may reduce or, in some instances, obviate the need for analgesics. Nonpharmacological interventions are also effective adjuncts to pharmacological pain management and they should be combined as frequently as possible. Nonpharmacological interventions alone should be used for only minor invasive procedures. For more invasive procedures, potent pharmacological analgesics must be used.

References

1. Stevens B, Anand KJ (2000) An overview of neonatal pain. In: Anand KJ, Stevens B, McGrath P (eds) Pain in neonates. Elsevier Science, Amsterdam, pp 1–7
2. Fitzgerald M (2000) Development of the peripheral and spinal pain system. In: Anand KJ, Stevens B, McGrath P (eds) Pain in neonates. Elsevier Science, Amsterdam, pp 9–21
3. Simons SH, van Dijk M, Anand KS et al (2003) Do we still hurt newborn babies? A prospective study of procedural pain and analgesia in neonates. Arch Pediatr Adolesc Med 157:1058–1064
4. Barker DP, Rutter N (1995) Exposure to invasive procedures in neonatal intensive care unit admissions. Arch Dis Child Fetal Neonatal Ed 72:F47–F48

5. Carbajal R, Rousset A, Marchand A et al (2007) Number of invasive procedures and corresponding analgesic therapy in neonates admitted to NICUs and PICUs: The EPIPPAIN Multicenter Study. Pediatric Academic Societies' Annual Meeting, 5–8 May 2007, Toronto, Canada. E-PAS2007:61:6281.3. Available at http://www.abstracts2view.com/pas/
6. Stevens B, Gibbins S, Franck LS (2000) Treatment of pain in the neonatal intensive care unit. Pediatr Clin North Am 47:633–650
7. Menon G, Anand K J, McIntosh N (1998) Practical approach to analgesia and sedation in the neonatal intensive care unit. Semin Perinatol 22:417–424
8. Harpin VA, Rutter N (1983) Making heel pricks less painful. Arch Dis Child 58:226–228
9. McIntosh N, van Veen L, Brameyer H (1994) Alleviation of the pain of heel prick in preterm infants. Arch Dis Child Fetal Neonatal Ed 70:F177–F181
10. Barker D, Latty B, Rutter N (1994) Heel blood sampling in preterm infants: which technique? Arch Dis Child Fetal Neonatal Ed 71:F206-F208
11. Paes B, Janes M, Vegh P et al (1993) A comparative study of heel-stick devices for infant blood collection. Am J Dis Child 147:346–348
12. Barker DP, Willetts B, Cappendijk VC, Rutter N (1996) Capillary blood sampling: should the heel be warmed? Arch Dis Child Fetal Neonatal Ed 74:F139–F140
13. Larsson BA, Tannfeldt G, Lagercrantz H, Olsson GL (1998) Venipuncture is more effective and less painful than heel lancing for blood tests in neonates. Pediatrics 101:882–886
14. Shah VS, Taddio A, Bennett S, Speidel BD (1997) Neonatal pain response to heel stick vs venepuncture for routine blood sampling. Arch Dis Child Fetal Neonatal Ed 77:F143–F144
15. Shah V, Ohlsson A (2004) Venepuncture versus heel lance for blood sampling in term neonates. Cochrane Database Syst Rev 4:CD001452
16. Blackburn S, Patteson D (1991) Effects of cycled light on activity state and cardiorespiratory function in preterm infants. J Perinat Neonatal Nurs 4:47–54
17. Mann N P, Haddow R, Stokes L et al (1986) Effect of night and day on preterm infants in a newborn nursery: randomised trial. Br Med J (Clin Res Ed) 293:1265–1267
18. Stevens B, Petryshen P, Hawkins J et al (1996) Developmental versus conventional care: a comparison of clinical outcomes for very low birth weight infants. Can J Nurs Res 28:97–113
19. Campos RG (1989) Soothing pain-elicited distress in infants with swaddling and pacifiers. Child Dev 60:781–792
20. Fearon I, Kisilevsky BS, Hains SM et al (1997) Swaddling after heel lance: age-specific effects on behavioral recovery in preterm infants. J Dev Behav Pediatr 18:222–232
21. Prasopkittikun T, Tilokskulchai F (2003) Management of pain from heel stick in neonates: an analysis of research conducted in Thailand. J Perinat Neonatal Nurs 17:304–312
22. Corff KE, Seideman R, Venkataraman PS et al (1995) Facilitated tucking: a nonpharmacologic comfort measure for pain in preterm neonates. J Obstet Gynecol Neonatal Nurs 24:143–147
23. Grunau R E, Linhares M B, Holsti L et al (2004) Does prone or supine position influence pain responses in preterm infants at 32 weeks gestational age? Clin J Pain 20:76–82
24. Field T, Goldson E (1984) Pacifying effects of nonnutritive sucking on term and preterm neonates during heelstick procedures. Pediatrics 74:1012–1015
25. Shiao SY, Chang YJ, Lannon H, Yarandi H (1997) Meta-analysis of the effects of nonnutritive sucking on heart rate and peripheral oxygenation: research from the past 30 years. Issues Compr Pediatr Nurs 20:11–24
26. Stevens B, Johnston C, Franck L et al (1999) The efficacy of developmentally sensitive interventions and sucrose for relieving procedural pain in very low birth weight neonates. Nurs Res 48:35–43
27. Corbo MG, Mansi G, Stagni A et al (2000) Nonnutritive sucking during heelstick procedures decreases behavioral distress in the newborn infant. Biol Neonate 77:162–167
28. Blass EM, Watt LB (1999) Suckling- and sucrose-induced analgesia in human newborns. Pain 83:611–623
29. Bellieni CV, Bagnoli F, Perrone S et al (2002) Effect of multisensory stimulation on analgesia in term neonates: a randomized controlled trial. Pediatr Res 51:460–463

30. Carbajal R, Chauvet X, Couderc S, Olivier-Martin M (1999) Randomised trial of analgesic effects of sucrose, glucose, and pacifiers in term neonates. BMJ 319:1393–1397
31. Pinelli J, Symington A, Ciliska D (2002) Nonnutritive sucking in high-risk infants: benign intervention or legitimate therapy? J Obstet Gynecol Neonatal Nurs 31:582–591
32. Blass EM, Hoffmeyer LB (1991) Sucrose as an analgesic for newborn infants. Pediatrics 87:215–218
33. Stevens B, Yamada J, Ohlsson A (2004) Sucrose for analgesia in newborn infants undergoing painful procedures. Cochrane Database Syst Rev 3:CD001069
34. Stevens B, Taddio A, Ohlsson A, Einarson T (1997) The efficacy of sucrose for relieving procedural pain in neonates – a systematic review and meta-analysis. Acta Paediatr 86:837–842
35. Johnston CC, Stremler R, Horton L, Friedman A (1999) Effect of repeated doses of sucrose during heel stick procedure in preterm neonates. Biol Neonate 75:160–166
36. Barr RG, Quek VS, Cousineau D et al (1994) Effects of intra-oral sucrose on crying, mouthing and hand-mouth contact in newborn and six-week-old infants. Dev Med Child Neurol 36:608–618
37. Allen KD, White DD, Walburn JN (1996) Sucrose as an analgesic agent for infants during immunization injections. Arch Pediatr Adolesc Med 150:270–274
38. Barr RG, Young SN, Wright JH et al (1995) "Sucrose analgesia" and diphtheria-tetanus-pertussis immunizations at 2 and 4 months. J Dev Behav Pediatr 16:220–225
39. Rogers AJ, Greenwald MH, Deguzman MA et al (2006) A randomized, controlled trial of sucrose analgesia in infants younger than 90 days of age who require bladder catheterization in the pediatric emergency department. Acad Emerg Med 13:617–622
40. Lewindon PJ, Harkness L, Lewindon N (1998) Randomised controlled trial of sucrose by mouth for the relief of infant crying after immunisation. Arch Dis Child 78:453–456
41. Ramenghi LA, Webb AV, Shevlin PM et al (2002) Intra-oral administration of sweet-tasting substances and infants' crying response to immunization: a randomized, placebo-controlled trial. Biol Neonate 81:163–169
42. Schechter NL, Zempsky WT, Cohen LL et al (2007) Pain reduction during pediatric immunizations: evidence-based review and recommendations. Pediatrics 119:e1184–1198
43. Barr RG, Pantel MS, Young SN et al (1999) The response of crying newborns to sucrose: is it a "sweetness" effect? Physiol Behav 66:409–417
44. Prevention and management of pain and stress in the neonate. American Academy of Pediatrics. Committee on Fetus and Newborn. Committee on Drugs. Section on Anesthesiology. Section on Surgery. Canadian Paediatric Society. Fetus and Newborn Committee. Pediatrics, 2000. 105:454–61
45. Royal Australasian College of Physicians, Paediatrics & Child Health Division (2005) Guideline Statement: Management of Procedure-related Pain in Neonates. Available at http://www.racp.edu.au [follow the links to Health Policy and Advocacy, then Paediatrics and Child Health]
46. Skogsdal Y, Eriksson M, Schollin J (1997) Analgesia in newborns given oral glucose. Acta Paediatr 86:217–220
47. Carbajal R, Lenclen R, Gajdos V et al (2002) Crossover trial of analgesic efficacy of glucose and pacifier in very preterm neonates during subcutaneous injections. Pediatrics 110(2 Pt 1):389–393
48. Guala A, Pastore G, Liverani M E et al (2001) Glucose or sucrose as an analgesic for newborns: a randomised controlled blind trial. Minerva Pediatr 53:271–274
49. Isik U, Ozek E, Bilgen H, Cebeci D (2000) Comparison of oral glucose and sucrose solutions on pain response in neonates. J Pain 1:275–278
50. Deshmukh LS, Udani RH (2002) Analgesic effect of oral glucose in preterm infants during venipuncture – a double-blind, randomized, controlled trial. J Trop Pediatr 48:138–141
51. Eriksson M, Finnström O (2004) Can daily repeated doses of orally administered glucose induce tolerance when given for neonatal pain relief? Acta Paediatr 93:246–249
52. Gibbins S, Stevens B, Hodnett E et al (2002) Efficacy and safety of sucrose for procedural pain relief in preterm and term neonates. Nurs Res 51:375–382

53. Johnston CC, Filion F, Snider L et al (2002) Routine sucrose analgesia during the first week of life in neonates younger than 31 weeks' postconceptional age. Pediatrics 110:523–528
54. Bellieni CV, Buonocore G, Nenci A et al (2001) Sensorial saturation: an effective analgesic tool for heel-prick in preterm infants: a prospective randomized trial. Biol Neonate 80:15–18
55. Gray L, Watt L, Blass EM (2000) Skin-to-skin contact is analgesic in healthy newborns. Pediatrics 105:e14
56. Johnston CC, Stevens B, Pinelli J et al (2003) Kangaroo care is effective in diminishing pain response in preterm neonates. Arch Pediatr Adolesc Med 157:1084–1088
57. Gray L, Miller LW, Philipp BL, Blass EM (2002) Breastfeeding is analgesic in healthy newborns. Pediatrics 109:590–593
58. Carbajal R, Veerapen S, Couderc S et al (2003) Analgesic effect of breast feeding in term neonates: randomised controlled trial. BMJ 326:13
59. Shendurnikar N, Gandhi K (2005) Analgesic effects of breastfeeding on heel lancing. Indian Pediatr 42:730–732
60. Phillips RM, Chantry CJ, Gallagher MP (2005) Analgesic effects of breast-feeding or pacifier use with maternal holding in term infants. Ambul Pediatr 5:359–364
61. Bilgen H, Ozek E, Cebeci D, Ors R (2001) Comparison of sucrose, expressed breast milk, and breast-feeding on the neonatal response to heel prick. J Pain 2:301–305
62. Gradin M, Finnstrom O, Schollin J (2004) Feeding and oral glucose – additive effects on pain reduction in newborns. Early Hum Dev 77:57–65
63. Blass EM, Miller LW (2001) Effects of colostrum in newborn humans: dissociation between analgesic and cardiac effects. J Dev Behav Pediatr 22:385–390
64. Bucher HU, Baumgartner R, Bucher N et al (2000) Artificial sweetener reduces nociceptive reaction in term newborn infants. Early Hum Dev 59:51–60
65. Ors R, Ozek E, Baysoy G et al (1999) Comparison of sucrose and human milk on pain response in newborns. Eur J Pediatr 158:63–66
66. Upadhyay A, Aggarwal R, Narayan S et al (2004) Analgesic effect of expressed breast milk in procedural pain in term neonates: a randomized, placebo-controlled, double-blind trial. Acta Paediatr 93:518–522
67. Uyan ZS, Ozek E, Bilgen H et al (2005) Effect of foremilk and hindmilk on simple procedural pain in newborns. Pediatr Int 47:252–257
68. Shah PS, Aliwalas LI, Shah V (2006) Breastfeeding or breast milk for procedural pain in neonates. Cochrane Database Syst Rev 3:CD004950
69. Kemper KJ, Danhauer SC (2005) Music as therapy. South Med J 98:282–288
70. Bo LK, Callaghan P (2000) Soothing pain-elicited distress in Chinese neonates. Pediatrics 105:E49
71. Butt ML, Kisilevsky BS (2000) Music modulates behaviour of premature infants following heel lance. Can J Nurs Res 31:17–39
72. Cignacco E, Hamers JP, Stoffel L et al (2007) The efficacy of non-pharmacological interventions in the management of procedural pain in preterm and term neonates. A systematic literature review. Eur J Pain 11:139–152

Chapter 11
Sensory Saturation: An Analgesic Method

C.V. Bellieni, M. Maffei and G. Buonocore

Until a few years ago, it was claimed that the word 'pain' was inappropriate for new-borns, as pain is a subjective experience that newborns, because of their age, cannot have [1], and until the 1980s opioids were rarely administered to newborns in the case of surgery [2]. We are now aware that newborns actually feel pain and that anesthesia reduces brain damage due to hypoxemia, hypertension, tachycardia, variations in heart rate, and increased intracranial pressure provoked by pain [3, 4], all of which are particularly dangerous in premature babies because of the immaturity of their cerebral vasoregulation [5].

Guidelines for the management of neonatal pain have been suggested [6–9], especially in connection with blood sampling, which is often performed by heel prick. To avoid the drawbacks of general and topical analgesics [10–15], non-pharmacologic methods of analgesia have been proposed. These include nonnutritional sucking [15] and instillation of glucose or other sweet liquids on the tongue [16, 17]; glucose is supposed to provide analgesia by stimulating incretion of β-endorphins [16, 18–20] through a preabsorption mechanism [21]. However, although the methods used have reduced the signs of pain perception, they have not eliminated them [22–27].

We recently developed a nonpharmacologic system to produce analgesia in new-borns during minor invasive procedures [28, 29]. It consists in giving stimuli (tactile, auditory, olfactory, and visual) during a painful minor procedure. These stimuli compete with the pain transmission to the central nervous system, and for this reason we call it "sensory saturation". We have shown that these stimuli are ineffective without the analgesic effect of oral sugar, but, when added to it, they greatly increase the analgesic effect of an oral sweet solution.

The main explanation of this effect is the so called "gate control theory" [30], according to which the brain is not a passive receiver of nociceptive input but can influence the information received, deciding whether or not it is important enough to record. Stimulation of sensory channels prevents nociceptive nerve impulses from getting through [31–33]. We studied this technique in 17 premature babies for whom it was clinically necessary to perform a heel prick five times. To determine which analgesic method was the most effective, we used a different one each of the five times. The order in which the different methods were used was randomized. Either no analgesia was attempted (control sample) or sucking, oral glucose with or without sucking, and

G. Buonocore, C.V. Bellieni (eds), *Neonatal Pain. Suffering, Pain and Risk of Brain Damage in the Fetus and Newborn,* © Springer 2008

sensory saturation were used for analgesic effect. The babies were filmed during the procedure. The Premature Infant Pain Profile (PIPP) was used to score pain as it is precise and takes into account gestational age, wakefulness, oxygen saturation, heart rate, and facial expressions. Without glucose, pain scores were high, but glucose alone had little analgesic effect. Glucose plus sucking was associated with a significantly lower pain score. However, with sensory saturation the babies did not feel pain. Glucose plus sucking reduced pain with respect to the control but did not eliminate it. We knew this from the literature: babies sucking sugar solution cry less, but they still cry a lot. In 1996, Abad showed that after oral administration of glucose during blood sampling, babies cried for 20 s during the 3-min observation period [34]. We repeated our study in 120 term babies and saw that with sensory saturation, term babies cried for an average of 2.8 s throughout the heel-prick procedure [28].

We also investigated the increase in intracranial pressure during acute pain and whether it was modified by sensory saturation. The instrument we used to measure intracranial pressure was the tonometer that oculists use to measure eye pressure. Measuring intracranial pressure by applying the tonometer to the anterior fontanel was validated in 1982 to assess intracranial pressure in babies with cranial drainage [35]. We studied 51 premature babies: one group was studied during blood sampling from the external jugular vein, a second during heel prick, and a third during heel prick with the aid of sensory saturation [36]. We measured intracranial pressure before and during the various samplings to see how much it increased: sensory saturation almost completely canceled out this increase.

Sensory saturation is not complex: when correctly explained it is easily learnt. Some examples can be seen at URL: http://www.euraibi.com. We recently showed that it can be easily performed by mothers with 5 min training as effectively as by experienced nurses [37]. It is worth remembering that the sign that the baby is ready to receive the prick without pain is his/her having rhythmic sucking, a sign that relaxation and distraction have been achieved.

As sensory saturation is more effective than oral sugar solution or sucking, it should be implemented as well as other methods which have shown their analgesic effectiveness (e.g. breastfeeding): newborns need not merely a drug or a "good technical procedure" during a painful event, but a human presence that accompanies, distracts, and comforts them.

References

1. De Lima J et al (1996) Infant and neonatal pain. BMJ 313:787
2. Beyer JE, DeGood DE, Ashley LC et al (1983) Patterns of postoperative analgesic use with adults and children following cardiac surgery. Pain 17:71–81
3. Anand KJ (1998) Clinical importance of pain and stress in preterm neonates. Biol Neonate 73:1–9
4. Stevens BJ, Johnston CC (1994) Physiological responses of premature infants to a painful stimulus. Nurs Res 43:226–231

5. Tsuji M, Saul P, du Plessis A et al (2000) Cerebral intravascular oxygenation corre-lates with mean arterial pressure in critically ill premature infants. Pediatrics 106:625–632
6. Anonymous (2000) Prevention and management of pain and stress in the neonate. Pediatrics 105:454–458
7. Spaeth JP, O'Hara IB, Kurth CD (1998) Anesthesia for the micropremie. Semin Perinatol 22:390–401
8. Stevens B, Gibbins S, Franck LS (2000) Treatment of pain in the neonatal intensive care unit. Pediatr Clin North Am 47:633–640
9. Carbajal R, Simon N (1995) Sédation et analgésie chez l'enfant. Arch Pédiatr 2:1089–1096
10. Jacqz-Aigrain E, Burtin P (1996) Clinical pharmacokinetics of sedatives in neonates. Clin Pharmacokinet 31:423–443
11. Levene M (1995) Pain relief and sedation during neonatal intensive care. Eur J Pediatr 54(Suppl 3):S22–S23
12. Law RMT, Halpern S, Martins RF et al (1996) Measurement of methemoglobin after EMLA analgesia for newborn circumcision. Biol Neonate 70:213–217
13. Gourrier E, Karoubi P, El Hanache A et al (1995) Utilisation de la crème EMLA chez le nouveau-né à terme et prématuré. Etude d'efficacité et de tolérance. Arch Pédiatr 2:1041–1046
14. Lemmen RJ, Semmekrot BA (1996) Muscle rigidity causing life-threatening hypercap-nia following fentanyl administration in a premature infant. Eur J Pediatr 155:1067
15. Blass EM, Watt LB (1999) Suckling and sucrose induced analgesia in human newborns. Pain 83:611–623
16. Blass EM, Fitzgerald E (1988) Milk-induced analgesia and comforting in 10-day-old rats: opioid mediation. Pharmacol Biochem Behav 29:9–3
17. Blass EM (1997) Milk-induced hypoalgesia in human newborns. Pediatrics 99:825–829
18. Balon-Perin S, Kolanowski J, Berbinschi A et al (1991) The effects of glucose ingestion and fasting on plasma immunoreactive beta-endorphin, adrenocorticotropic hormone and cortisol in obese subjects. J Endocrinol Invest 14:919–925
19. Tropeano G, Lucisano A, Liberale I et al (1994) Insulin, C-peptide, androgens and endor-phin response to oral glucose in patients with polycystic ovary syndrome. J Clin Endocrinol Metab 78:305–309
20. Shide DJ, Blass EEM (1989) Opioid-like effects in intraoral infusions of corn oil and polycose on stress reactions in 10-day-old rats. Behav Neurosi 103:1168–1175
21. Ramenghi LA, Evans DJ, Levene MI (1999) 'Sucrose analgesia': absorptive mechanism or taste perception? Arch Dis Child Fetal Neonatal Ed 80:F146–F147
22. Abad F, Diaz NM, Domenech E et al (1996) Oral sweet solution reduces pain-related behaviour in preterm infants. Acta Paediatr 85:854–858
23. Bucher HU, Moser T, Von Siebental K et al (1995) Sucrose reduces pain reaction to heel lancing in preterm infants: a placebo-controlled, randomized and masked study. Pediatr Res 38:332–335
24. Stevens B, Johnston C, Franck L et al (1999) The efficacy of developmentally sensitive interventions and sucrose for relieving procedural pain in very low birth weight neonates. Nurs Res 48:35–43
25. Johnston CC, Stremler RL, Stevens BJ, Horton LJ (1997) Effectiveness of oral sucrose and simulated rocking on pain response in preterm neonates. Pain 72:193–199
26. McIntosh N, van Veen L, Brameyer H (1994) Alleviation of the pain of heel prick in preterm infants. Arch Dis Child 70:F177–F181
27. Ramenghi L, Wood CM, Griffith GC, Levene MI (1996) Reduction of pain response in premature infants using intraoral sucrose. Arch Dis Child 74:F126–F128
28. Bellieni CV, Bagnoli F, Perrone S et al (2002) Effect of multisensory stimulation on anal-gesia in term neonates: a randomised controlled trial. Pediatr Res 51:460–463
29. Bellieni CV, Buonocore G, Nenci A et al (2001) Sensorial saturation: an effective anal-gesic tool for heel-prick in preterm infants: a prospective randomized trial. Biol Neonate 80:15–18

30. Lindahl S (1997) Calming minds or killing pain in newborn infants? Acta Paediatr 86:787–788
31. Melzack R, Wall PD (1965) Pain mechanisms: a new theory. Science 150:971–979
32. Wall PD (1978) The gate control theory of pain mechanism. A re-examination and re-statement. Brain 101:1–18
33. Melzack R (1999) From the gate to the neuromatrix. Pain 6:S121–S126
34. Abad F, Diaz NM, Domenech E et al (1996) Oral sweet solution reduces pain-related behaviour in preterm infants. Acta Paediatr 85:854–848
35. Easa D, Tran A, Bingham W (1983) Noninvasive intracranial pressure measurement in the newborn. Am J Dis Child 137:332–335
36. Bellieni CV, Burroni A, Perrone S et al (2003) Intracranial pressure during procedural pain. Biol Neonate 84:202–205
37. Bellieni CV, Cordelli DM, Marchi S et al (2007) Sensorial saturation for neonatal analgesia. Clin J Pain 23:219–221

Chapter 12
Pharmacologic Analgesia in the Newborn

A.M. Guadagni

There is increasing evidence that neuroanatomic and neuroendocrine components for the perception and transmission of painful stimuli are fully developed in the newborn even when preterm. Incomplete myelination only means slower transmission. Pain in the newborn increases heart rate, mean airway pressure, O_2 consumption, and levels of catecholamines, corticosteroids, and glucagons; decreases arterial O_2 saturation; produces acidosis, hyperglycemia, and pulmonary hypertension; and increases susceptibility to infections and intraventricular hemorrhage (preterms) [1, 2]. Untreated pain may in fact exacerbate injury, increase the incidence of neurological handicap, lead to infection, prolong hospitalization, and may even lead to death [3, 4].

Major advances in neurobiology, from molecular studies to imaging the cortex of the brain, show the complex integration of nerve cell activity and have brought about a fundamental change in attitude and expectations regarding the control of pain [5]. Hospitalized newborns are subjected to many invasive procedures as part of their medical care: care-giving (bathing, diaper changing, feeding, placing of orogastric and nasogastric tubes, weighing, measuring); diagnostic (heel, venous and arterial puncture, radiography, ultrasonography, lumbar puncture, bronchoscopy and esophagoscopy, eye examination for retinopathy of prematurity); and therapeutic (insertion of chest tubes and other drainages, tracheal intubation and mechanical ventilation, bronchoalveolar lavage, endotracheal suction, peripheral and central line insertion, cannulation for extracorporeal membrane oxygenation and continuous arterovenous haemodialysis, surgery, and postoperative management).

Today healthcare professionals expect to control pain by using preventive and active strategies including nonpharmacological and pharmacological treatment of neonatal pain. The Association of European Scientists has promulgated standard-of-care guidelines and/or position statements regarding neonatal pain management, to increase long-term quality of life [6].

Comfort Measures

The suffering of neonates can be avoided. Quieting techniques are a useful way to help control pain response in the neonate.

G. Buonocore, C.V. Bellieni (eds), *Neonatal Pain. Suffering, Pain and Risk of Brain Damage in the Fetus and Newborn*, © Springer 2008

- Always minimize discomfort and limit painful procedures.
- Give the neonate glucose or sucrose 10–15% to suck [7–9].
- Sensory saturation (massage, voice, eye contact, perfume and sucrose) is also effective [10].

Local Analgesia

Topical anesthetics provide analgesia for minor invasive procedures by preventing the transmission of noxious stimuli either at the peripheral receptor site or at the spinal cord.

Bupivacaine and *lidocaine* are the two drugs most commonly used for local infiltration in solution (0.5–1%), in painful procedures. Bupivacaine is longer acting but more cardiotoxic than lidocaine. Toxicity is determined by its absorption in the systemic circulation.

Bupivacaine and ropivacaine are drugs used for infusion with a peridural catheter in 0.25% solution. If they are administered using regional techniques, stress responses are significantly decreased, the need for postoperative ventilation may be avoided or shortened, and intestinal motility recovers more quickly. Regional techniques have been investigated for safety and efficacy in neonates and infants. Adding opioids to local anesthetic epidural infusions may have the benefit of reducing the dose of local anesthetic required to produce adequate analgesia, thereby decreasing the risk of toxicity. Varying opinion exists among pediatric anesthesia practitioners regarding the relative risks and benefits of using opioids either exclusively or in combination with local anesthetics in epidural infusions, compared to local anesthetic-only epidural infusions.

EMLA (euthetic mixture of local anesthetic) is an emulsion containing prilocaine and lidocaine. Continuous or repeated use may cause methemoglobinemia because methemoglobin reductase is deficient in the newborn. This does not appear to be a problem in premature neonates if it is used only once in a day. The recommended dose is 1–2 g 60 min before procedure, and the site must be covered with a water-impermeable dressing [11, 12]. EMLA is not recommended for heel prick because it produces local vasoconstriction.

General Analgesia

Nonnarcotic Drugs

Acetaminophen and nonsteroidal anti-inflammatory drugs can be helpful in providing mild to moderate analgesia. They produce analgesia for moderate pain but

when given alone do not relieve surgical pain [13, 14]. Dosages are:
- Acetaminophen 10–15 mg/kg every 6 h p.o.; 20–30 mg/kg every 6 h p.r. (overdose may cause hepatotoxicity).
- Ibuprofen 5–10 mg/kg every 6 h p.o. (gastric irritant, must be used with caution in neonates with neonatal entero colitis).

Sedatives used in the newborn are *midazolam* and *lorazepam*. They can help decrease agitation, improve comfort, and increase the effect of narcotics, but do not by themselves provide analgesia. Dosages are:
- Midazolam 0.05–0.1 mg/kg i.v. and 0.02–0.06 mg/kg/h.
- Lorazepam 0.05–0.1 mg/kg i.v. or p.o. every 4–8 h.

Narcotic Drugs

Narcotic drugs are opiates (morphine) and opioids (fentanyl, sufentanil, remifentanil, etc.). They are recognized as the standard drug for pain relief in major invasive procedures (artificial ventilation, surgical procedures, chest tube placement). Recognition of their limitations has, however, enabled a broad reappraisal of the indications for opioid treatment. These can be classified as either μ or k depending on the receptor subtype at which they exert their action, with a similar mechanism in each case.

Absorption, metabolism, distribution, and clearance of drugs in the neonate differ from those in the older child. The target steady-state concentration is influenced by gestational age, age since birth, and weight, and also by the fraction of drug bound to plasma proteins. There are differences also in onset and duration of action, and important differences also relating to the modality of administration (intravenous, continuous infusion, oral, rectal). The goal of the treatment is to achieve and maintain a free drug concentration at the site of action that will produce the maximum desired effect with a minimal risk of toxicity. Opioids produce adverse effects that can be minimized by appropriate drug selection and dosing. Respiratory depression, hypotension, glottic and chest wall rigidity, constipation, seizures, sedation, and bradycardia are well described.

The most commonly used drugs to treat or prevent pain are morphine and fentanyl. They decrease cortisolemia [15], decrease stress [1, 16], and produce better ventilator synchrony [17], oxygenation [18], and blood pressure stability [19].

Morphine remains the gold standard for comparison of all other opioids. Morphine is an extract of opium and a standard opioid analgesic for all ages including neonates; it has induced histamine release, pruritus, urinary retention, and seizures (reported in the newborn at "standard" intravenous doses). Hypotension and bradycardia are part of the histamine response to morphine and are associated with rapid intravenous bolus administration. Morphine is 70–80 times less potent than fentanyl and produced less tolerance and withdrawal effects than fentanyl.

Fentanyl is a synthetic opioid with a large postulated effect on the μ-receptor. Fentanyl has a wide margin of safety and beneficial effects on hemodynamic stability [20]. It has a rapid onset and short duration of action. Chest wall and glottis rigidity are adverse effects with high bolus dosing (>5 μg/kg), but may occur even with low doses (1–2 μg/kg) if infusion is too rapid. The short duration of action (<60 min) is because of its distribution (high lipid solubility).

Remifentanil is a new opioid selective μ-receptor agonist with a higher potency than alfentanil. The metabolism is independent of liver and renal function and reacts with nonspecific esterase in tissue and erythrocytes; carbonic acid is excreted through the kidneys. Intravenous remifentanil doses of 0.25 μg/kg per minute appear to be safe and effective in neonates [21, 22], but data concerning the use of remifentanil in this group are few. The decision as to which opioid to use depends on the type of underlying pathology in the neonate, the type of procedures intended, the duration of treatment, and the experience of the neonatal intensive care unit.

Drugs used for endotracheal intubation are:
– Atropine 0.02 μg/kg i.v.
– Fentanyl 0.5–2 μg/kg i.v. in 3–5 min.
– Succinylcholine 1–2 mg/kg i.v..
– Remifentanil 0.1–0.25 μg/kg per minute as a continuous infusion.
Drugs used for mechanical ventilation are:
– Morphine 50–100 μg/kg i.v. or 10.50 μg/kg/h.
– Fentanyl 0.5–3 μg/kg i.v. in 30 min, or 0.5–2 μg/kg/h.
– Remifentanil: 0.1–0.25 μg/kg per minute as a continuous infusion.

The side effects of treatment are constipation and urinary retention (opioids), respiratory depression (opioids), histamine release and bronchoconstriction (morphine), chest wall and glottis rigidity (fentanyl), tolerance and withdrawal effects (opioids), and myoclonic movements (midazolam).

The duration of opioid receptor occupancy is important for the development of tolerance and dependence, which occurs when the total opioids dosage is greater than 1.6 mg/kg or infusion for more than 5 days. The infusion modality is also very important: continuous infusion of opioids may produce tolerance more rapidly than an intravenous bolus. To minimize withdrawal syndrome, dosage must be decreased by 20% in the first 24 h and by 10% every 12 h thereafter [24].

If respiratory depression occurs, naloxone 10 μg/kg may be given intramuscularly or intravenously. Naloxone also antagonizes endorphin effects.

Future Perspectives

Future developments will include:
– Use of regional analgesia technique.
– Sequential rotation of analgesics.

– Bolus vs. continuous infusion of opioids.
– Use of new opioids (remifentanil).
– Addition of ultra-low doses of opioid antagonists (naloxone).
– Use of noncompetitive NMDA antagonists (methadone-dextromethorphan) [25].

In conclusion, analgesia and sedation represent an important component of the comprehensive optimal management of the newborn; however, caution must be exercised because of possible side effects and/or complications of treatment. New drugs and novel approaches are recommended to be used, but tested before they are introduced into routine clinical practice.

References

1. Anand KJ, Hickey PR (1987) Pain and its effects in the human neonate and fetus. N Engl J Med 317:1321–1329
2. Barker DP, Rutter N (1995) Exposure to invasive procedures in neonatal intensive care admissions. Arch Dis Child 72:F47–F48
3. Anand KJS, Barton BA, McIntosh N et al (1999) Analgesia and sedation in preterm neonates who require ventilatory support. Results from the NOPAIN trial. Arch Pediatr Adolesc Med 153:331–338
4. Barker DP, Rutter N (1996) Stress, severity of illness, and outcome in ventilated preterm infants. Arch Dis Child Fetal Neonatal Ed 75:F187–F190
5 Dubner R, Gold M (1999) The neurobiology of pain. Proc Natl Acad Sci USA 96:7627-7630
6. Anand KJS, International Evidence-Based Group for Neonatal Pain (2001) Consensus statement for the prevention and management of pain in the newborn. Arch Pediatr Adolesc Med 155:173–180
7. Blass EM (1991) Sucrose as an analgesic for newborn infants. Pediatrics 87:215
8. Bucher HW (1995) Sucrose reduce pain reaction to heel lancing in preterm infants. Pediatr Res 38:332–335
9. Stevens B (1997) The efficacy of sucrose for relieving procedural pain in neonates. Arch Pediatr 86:837–842
10. Bellieni CV, Bagnoli F, Perrone S et al (2002) Effect of multisensory stimulation on analgesia in term neonates: a randomized controlled trial. Pediatr Res 51:460–463
11. Gourrier E (1995) Use of EMLA cream in premature and full-term newborn infants. Study of efficacy and tolerance. Arch Pediatr 2:1041–1046
12. Taddio A (1996) Safety of lidocaine-prilocaine cream in preterm and full term neonates. Pediatr Res 39:80A
13. Autret E, Dutertre JP, Breteau M et al (1993) Pharmacokinetics of paracetamol in neonate and infant after administration of proparacetamol chlorhydrate. Dev Pharmacol Ther 20:129–134
14. Shah V, Taddio A, Ohlsson A (1998) Randomised controlled trial of paracetamol for heel prick pain in neonates. Arch Dis Child 79:F209–F211
15. Orsini AJ (1996) Routine use of fentanyl infusion for pain and stress reduction in infants with respiratory distress. J Pediatr 129:140–145
16. Quinn MW, Wild J, Dean HG et al (1993) Randomised double-blind controlled trial of effect of morphine on catecholamine concentrations in ventilated preterm babies. Lancet 342:324–327
17. Dyke MP, Kohan R, Evans S (1995) Morphine increases synchronous ventilation in preterm infants. J Paediatr Child Health 31:176–179
18. Pokela ML (1994) Pain relief can reduce hypoxemia in distressed neonates during routine treatment procedures. Pediatrics 93:379–383

19. Goldstein RF, Brazy JE (1991) Narcotic sedation stabilizes arterial blood pressure fluc-
    tuations in sick premature infants. J Perinatol 11:365–371
20. Saarenmaa E, Huttunen P, Leppäluoto J et al (1999) Advantages of fentanyl over mor-
    phine in analgesia for ventilated newborn infants after birth: a randomized trial. J Pediatr
    134:144–150
21. Davis PJ, Galinkin J, McGowan FX et al (2001) A randomised multicenter study of
    remifentaniyl compared with halothane in neonates and infants undergoing pyloromy-
    otomy. Anesth Analg 93:1380–1386
22. Chiaretti A, Pietrini D, Piastra M et al (2000) Safety and efficacy of remifentaniyl in cran-
    iosynostosis repair in children less than 1 year old. Pediatr Neurosurg 33:83–88
23. Barrington KJ (1998) Premedication for neonatal intubations. Am J Perinatol 15:213–216
24. Suresh S, Anand KJS (2001) Opioid tolerance in neonates: a state of the art review. Pediatr
    Anaesth 11:511–521
25. Yeh GC, Tao PL, Chen JY et al (2002) Dextromethorphan attenuates morphine withdrawal
    syndrome in neonatal rats passively exposed to morphine. Eur J Pharmacol 453:197–202

Chapter 13
Physical Stress Risk Agents in Incubators

R. Sisto

Introduction

Physical risks in incubators mainly relate to noise and electromagnetic radiation exposure. The special vulnerability of neonates, associated with the development of their central nervous system and sensory apparatuses, suggests that particular care should be taken in monitoring their exposure to risk agents. The present chapter provides a brief introduction to these topics.

Noise Exposure

Noise exposure may be quantified according to the objective physical characteristics of the associated acoustic signal, or according to the level of subjective loudness and annoyance reported by the listener. Both aspects are relevant to understanding the effects of noise exposure on humans, and therefore a short introduction to these two complementary points of view seems useful.

Physical and Psychological Nature of Acoustic Noise

Physics

Any medium characterized by inertia and elasticity may propagate oscillatory waves. An acoustic wave is a perturbation of pressure and of the velocity field associated with spatially coherent oscillatory motion of the medium (a fluid, like air or water, a solid body, or a plasma) propagating through it at the speed of sound. In air, acoustic waves propagate pressure perturbations that are small fluctuations around the equilibrium atmospheric pressure value (for example, the pressure fluctuation associated with the sound level of typical noisy classrooms amounts to approximately one millionth of the atmospheric pressure).

G. Buonocore, C.V. Bellieni (eds), *Neonatal Pain. Suffering, Pain and Risk of Brain Damage in the Fetus and Newborn*, © Springer 2008

Acoustic waves with a frequency in the audible range (20 Hz to 20 kHz) give rise to sound perception in the human. Infrasonic and ultrasonic waves do not cause auditory perception. Infrasound may be perceived as an annoying vibration, while ultrasounds may be harmful for humans.

Acoustic noise is a stochastic signal, whose evolution in time is characterized by absence of phase coherence, while its spectrum may also show a resonant shape, according to the geometry of the environment. Mathematically, due to complete lack of phase coherence, a stochastic signal is completely characterized by its autocorrelation function, or, equivalently, by its power spectrum, which is the Fourier transform of the autocorrelation function.

Acoustic or sound pressure level (SPL) is expressed in decibels (dB SPL), and defined as:

$$L(dB) = 10 \log_{10} \left(\frac{p^2}{p_{o^2}} \right) \tag{1}$$

where p is the acoustic pressure, expressed in pascals (Pa), and p_0 is the standard reference pressure $p_0 = 20 \ \mu Pa$. The equivalent sound level is the mean square value of acoustic pressure calculated over a time interval T:

$$L_{eq}(dB) = 10 \log_{10} \frac{1}{T} \int_0^T \frac{p(t)^2}{p_{o^2}} dt . \tag{2}$$

The equivalent level L_{eq} is the level of a hypothetical constant noise that would produce, over the time interval T, the same acoustic energy as the phenomenon under consideration.

Psychoacoustics

In psychoacoustics, "noise" is a sound characterized by absence of semantic content, and that produces annoyance in the listener. Both the physical intensity and the semantic content of the acoustic signal contribute to the subjective sensation level of annoyance. The subjective evaluation of the sound intensity is defined in psychoacoustics as loudness. Isophonic curves provide a representation of the psychoacoustic hearing sensitivity as a function of frequency. These curves, for each frequency, connect sound levels corresponding to the same loudness sensation of a 1 kHz tone of a given level.

The parameter commonly used to evaluate the risk associated with exposure to noise is the A-weighted equivalent sound level: $L_{A,eq}$. The A-weighting curve $A(f)$ approaches the ear sensitivity at the sound level of 40 dB, i.e., it equalizes the sound spectrum according to the different sensitivity of the ear at different frequencies at a level of 40 dB. For higher sound levels, which are relevant to the noise exposure issue, other weighting curves have been computed, but A-weighting is commonly used independently of the noise level, as a standard practice. The A-weighted sound pressure level is given by:

$$L_{A.eq}(dBA) = 10\log_{10}\left(\sum_k 10^{0.1L_{f(k)}+A_{f(k)}}\right)$$ (3)

Effects of Exposure to Noise

Auditory Effects

High levels of noise are responsible for hearing loss. A correlation has been well established between noise level, exposure duration, and hearing loss [1]. International Standard curves also take into account physiological hearing loss associated with aging, which is obviously not present in babies.

The risk of damage to the auditory system starts at sound levels of the order of 78–80 dBA (the "A" denotes use of the A-weighting filter). The inner ear is the most sensitive part of the auditory system. A sophisticated feedback system between the outer hair cells (OHCs) and the peripheral nervous system (at the brainstem level) provides active nonlinear amplification of the transverse vibration of the basilar membrane, which is responsible for the astounding hearing capability of humans in terms of perception threshold and frequency discrimination. The feedback mediated by the OHCs performs as an active filter, amplifying the cochlear response by narrowing the bandwidth of the detector. As a consequence, low threshold and good frequency resolution are closely related to each other. Unfortunately, OHCs are particularly sensitive to noise exposure. Above noise levels of 100–110 dBA, acute OHC damage effects can cause permanent hearing impairment, but OHCs show generally a good capability of recovering their functionality after acute exposure if they have enough time to do so. A more subtle risk is associated with chronic exposure to much lower levels of noise (as low as 80 dBA), which can cause permanent damage of the OHCs if recovery cannot be fully reached before the next noise exposure.

Nonauditory Effects

The effects of noise on human health show that noise, even at low levels, interacts with the organism in a complex way, also giving rise to nonauditory effects [2]. The nonauditory effects of noise, such as the annoyance effect, can induce psychological and somatic disturbances which can interfere with personal feeling and health, interpersonal relations, and so on. The sound levels that may induce annoyance can be very low. The most important nonauditory effects relate to cardiovascular diseases, sleep disturbances, and performance at work; direct effects on psychopathology are still controversial.

Noise Sources in Incubators

Typical Noise Levels in Incubators

Noise levels in incubators from various sources under different conditions were evaluated by Bellieni et al. [3]. Here, we summarize some of the main results of this study.

The main sources of noise are:
– Incubator engine (continuous)
– Opening and closing portholes (transient)
– Temperature alarm (occasional, short duration)
– Baby crying (may be frequent, unpredictable duration)

The noise levels found by the authors are summarized in Table 1. A typical background noise of 50 dBA can be found when the incubator is on. This is very high compared with the background noise measured the incubator is switched off: 34–36 dBA. The noise criteria adopted by the International Organization for Standardization (ISO) to prevent annoyance recommend noise levels for bedrooms or hospitals in the range of 25–35 dBA. Noise levels in the range 45–50 dBA exceed tolerability criteria established to prevent sleeping annoyance.

Reverberating and Resonant Characteristics of Incubators

As Table 1 shows, the greatest source of noise in the incubator is the cry of the neonate himself (noise levels above 80 dBA). The incubator is a highly reverberating acoustic environment, which amplifies the sounds produced inside it. As a con-

Table 1   Noise levels from various sources under different conditions. (From [3])

Measurement conditions	Noise level L_{eq} (dBA)		
	Open hood	Closed hood without sound absorber	Closed hood with sound absorber
Background noise, incubator OFF	36–37	34–36	33–35
Background noise, incubator ON	46–47	48–50	48–50
Opening and closing portholes	70–71	73–74	70–71
Temperature alarm	58–59	56–57	50–51
Baby crying	81–83	84–87	82–85

sequence, sounds originating inside the incubators produce noise levels at the neonate ear that typically exceed by about 3 dB the levels that would be produced by the same source in the open. Moreover, the geometry and size of the incubator are such that the incubator behaves as a resonating cavity for acoustic waves for several frequencies in the audible range. This causes development of persistent standing waves that can cause both hearing damage and annoyance.

Crying Distortion

The reverberating and resonating characteristics of the incubators are responsible for acoustic distortion phenomena. In particular, when the baby is crying its voice is heard amplified and distorted at the neonate ear position. These phenomena were analyzed by Bellieni et al. [3]. In their study an acoustic amplification–distortion index was calculated in each frequency band (thirds of octave) using the following expression:

$$Df = L_c - L_a, \tag{4}$$

where L_c is the sound level at the frequency f, measured within closed Plexiglas walls and L_a is the corresponding level measured without Plexiglas walls. Figure 1 shows the crying spectra inside the incubator in different environmental conditions.

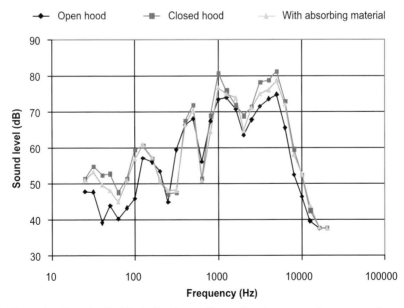

Fig. 1   Noise distortion inside the incubator. Comparison between noise spectra of neonate crying in different conditions of the incubator. (From [3])

Testing the Neonate Auditory System

Objective Diagnostic Tools

The neonate acoustic spectral sensitivity curve is not well established, because psychoacoustic techniques are not suitable for noncollaborating subjects such as neonates. However, objective techniques exist, from which it is possible to gain information about auditory function in neonates. Objective techniques include electrocochleography and measurement of acoustic brainstem response (ABR), steady-state ABR, and otoacoustic emissions (OAEs). Electrocochleography is a sensitive but rather invasive technique, requiring direct access to the cochlea by needle electrodes. ABR techniques require rather long averaging times, due to the low signal level, to reach a good signal-to-noise ratio, and are perturbed by the movements of the subject. Steady-state ABR techniques have been significantly improved in the last years, but are still affected by rather large uncertainties.

OAEs are acoustic signals which can be measured in the ear canal, in the presence (evoked OAEs) or absence (spontaneous OAEs, or SOAEs) of an external acoustic stimulus, as a consequence of activation of the OHCs' feedback system. Figure 2 shows a typical spectrum of spontaneous OAEs of a neonate. The high level of the peaks is notable.

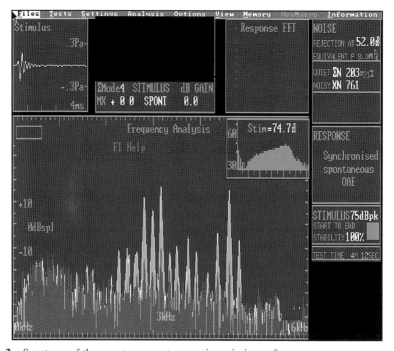

Fig. 2   Spectrum of the spontaneous otoacoustic emissions of a neonate

Evoked OAEs are classified according to the stimulus used to elicit them. Several different techniques are currently available. A main distinction is made between transient evoked OAEs (TEAOEs) and OAEs evoked by pure tones (stimulus-frequency OAEs, SFOAEs) or by two tones (distortion product OAEs, DPOAEs) [4].

Hearing Functionality and OAEs

As mentioned above, the nonlinear amplification active feedback mechanism providing the high sensitivity and sharp frequency resolution of the auditory system is localized in the cochlea, particularly in the OHCs, and OHCs are the first part of the auditory system to be damaged by high levels of noise exposure. The functionality of the cochlear active filter is also a necessary condition for the production of otoacoustic emissions, whose characteristics are very sensitive to small variations of the cochlear filter parameters. In fact, according to cochlear models of the OAE generation, the excitation level of the basilar membrane, which is strongly amplified by the active feedback mechanism, is directly related to the level of the OAEs. Therefore the sensitivity of hearing is correlated to the OAE levels.

Cochlear Tuning and OAEs

Another psychoacoustic characteristic of hearing, frequency discrimination capability, is related to measurable OAE parameters, namely the OAE characteristic delay times, which are often defined as latencies.

In psychoacoustics, cochlear tuning is the ability to discriminate sounds of different frequency, and it is measured using masking techniques. These techniques measure the variation of the perception threshold for a given frequency tone, as the frequency band of a masking noise signal approaches that frequency, identifying a critical band, which defines the frequency resolution of hearing.

In physics, cochlear tuning is related to the sharpness of the tonotopic cochlear filter, which is reflected in the activation pattern of the basilar membrane. Direct measurements of the basilar membrane frequency response have shown that the membrane's excitation pattern has a typical resonant shape. For each place x in the cochlea, the maximum basilar membrane displacement is given by its characteristic frequency $CF(x)$, with $CF(x)$ being an exponential function [5]. The width of the frequency response curve around $CF(x)$, or, equivalently, the width of the excitation pattern due to a single frequency $CF(x)$ around its tonotopic place x, is an increasing function of the stimulus level, and a direct measure of the frequency resolution of hearing.

Moleti and Sisto [6] demonstrated that it is also possible to estimate cochlear tuning for noncollaborating subjects, such as neonates, using a new technique based on time–frequency analysis of OAEs. The slowing down of each frequency component of the traveling wave approaching its tonotopic place is a function of the sharpness of the corresponding cochlear filter, and, therefore, cochlear tuning may be estimated from time-frequency measurements of the TEOAE latency, or from measurements of the phase-gradient delay of SFOAEs [7]. As is shown in Fig. 3, these OAE measurements show that the average neonate tuning curve is significantly higher than the adult curve, suggesting higher noise vulnerability in neonates. In fact, high effectiveness of the cochlear filter for intense signals could be associated with lower effectiveness of the self-defense efferent feedback mechanism protecting the ear from intense noise [6]. Other authors have used DPOAE tuning curves to reach the conclusion that immaturity of the efferent system reduces protection of the hearing system from intense noise in babies [8]. Recently, studies on premature neonates have shown that OAE latency is higher in preterm than in full-term neonates, which would accord with the above interpretations.

For the above reasons, neonates could be particularly vulnerable to noise, and among them, preterm neonates, which are more commonly exposed for quite a long time to the noisy incubator environment, could be the most vulnerable.

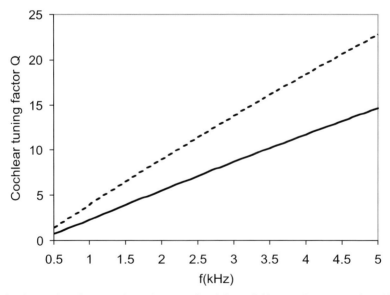

Fig. 3 Comparison between the tuning curve in adults (*solid line*) and neonates (*dotted line*), derived from otoacoustic emission latency measurements

Exposure to Electromagnetic Fields

Physical Nature of Electromagnetic Waves

An electromagnetic field consists of variable electric and magnetic fields that excite each other through their time variations. Such variable fields are generated by accelerated charges and variable currents. For oscillating sources, the period of oscillation $T = 1/f$ is related to the wavelength λ by the relation $\lambda = cT$ (or $\lambda = c/f$).

Electromagnetic radiation from a dipole source consists of several contributions, with different dependence on the distance from the source, with terms going as λ/r and $(\lambda/r)^2$, $(\lambda/r)^3$. Only the term with the λ/r dependence propagates energy radiating from the source, as for the others the time-averaged flux of the Poynting vector over a closed surface is null. The λ/r term is associated with electromagnetic radiation propagation, and it is dominant at distances much larger than the wavelength (far field). At great distances from the source ($r \gg \lambda$), the electromagnetic fields propagate at the speed of light as electromagnetic waves.

For visible radiation at macroscopic distances the far-field approximation is obviously correct, but for microwave and radio waves the other terms cannot be neglected, and become dominant.

At short distances from the source ($r \ll \lambda$) the near-field terms are dominant, which are time-modulated versions of the static dipole fields, which do not transmit any energy flux across a closed surface. For low-frequency electromagnetic fields, the near-field condition typically holds; for example, for $f = 1000$ Hz, $\lambda = 300$ km.

Interaction of Electromagnetic Fields with Biological Systems

Nonionizing Radiation and the Role of Frequency

Nonionizing radiation is characterized by the fact that the single photon energy, which is related to frequency by the relation $E = hf$, is not sufficient for ionizing a single atom or molecule. The quantum nature of the interaction between radiation and matter implies indeed that the single photon energy must exceed a well-defined threshold to excite or ionize an atom.

Frequency is the main physical parameter that influences the interaction between electromagnetic field and biological systems. A distinction is usually made between extremely low frequency (ELF, between 0 and 300 Hz), low frequency (VLF-LF, between 300 Hz and 300 kHz), radiofrequency (RF, between 300 kHz and 300 MHz) and microwave (MW, between 300 MHz and 300 GHz) radiation. At low frequency, the main effect of interaction is associated with the electrical current density (A/m^2) induced in the tissues. The induced current density is the physical quantity used to describe thresholds for acute effects and exposure limits. At frequencies above 100 kHz, the main interaction effect is the local heating of tissues. In this case, the physical parameter used to describe the effect threshold is the specific absorption rate (SAR), which is the electromagnetic power absorbed per unit mass (W/kg).

The development of the human being from conception to adulthood is continuous, but the prenatal period and the early stages of newborn development are the ones in which important changes take place in a short time. Therefore, like other risk agents, exposure to nonionizing radiation may be especially harmful for children, and particularly for neonates. Special attention should be given to the central nervous system and the hematopoietic and immune system, which are still under development, and particularly vulnerable, in neonates.

Acute Effects of Electromagnetic Fields

Acute effects are deterministic effects, with a typical induction threshold. The safety standards specify exposure limits both in terms of dosimetric quantities, such as induced current density or SAR, and in terms of maximum permissible amplitude of magnetic and electric fields (reference limits). The exposure limits for electric and magnetic field amplitude given by the International Commission on Non-Ionizing Radiation Protection (ICNIRP) to prevent acute effects at 50 Hz for the general population are, respectively:

$$E_{th} = 5000 \frac{V}{m}, \quad B_{th} = 100 \mu T. \tag{5}$$

Electromagnetic Fields: Long-Term Effects

The problem of possible long-term effects due to chronic exposure to low-intensity electromagnetic fields is quite a complex one [9]. The epidemiologic and experimental research carried on in recent years does not generally support the hypothesis of long-term effects due to chronic exposure to low-intensity fields. Nevertheless, some epidemiologic studies [10] have shown an association between residential exposure to ELF fields and increased risk increase of childhood leukemia, and a possible effect has been hypothesized for brain cancer. On the basis of these studies the International Agency for Research on Cancer (IARC), in June 2001, decided to classify the ELF fields as possibly carcinogenic (2B group) for humans. (IARC classification: 1, agent is carcinogenic for humans; 2A, agent is probably carcinogenic for humans; 2B, agent is possibly carcinogenic for humans.)

Electromagnetic Fields in Incubators

Some authors [11] reported the level of exposure to extremely low electromagnetic fields in transport incubators, and compared them to those typical of hospital incu-

Table 2 Maximum extremely low frequency (ELF) magnetic field in incubators. (From [11])

	Max B (μT)*
Transport incubator	35.7
Standard incubator	8.8

* Magnetic field maximum amplitude

bators. Because of their smaller size, the portable units are characterized by a shorter distance between the electric components and the neonate bed. As a consequence, the level of exposure is significantly higher in transport incubators (Table 2). These values are quite high, compared with the exposure to domestic ELF sources, and they are also close to the ICNIRP reference levels for population exposure to prevent acute effects (100 μT at 50 Hz). The authors showed that it is easy to reduce the exposure significantly simply by raising the mattress by 10 cm.

References

1. International Standard ISO 1999 (1990) Acoustics – determination of occupational noise exposure and estimation of noise-induced hearing impairment. International Organization for Standardization, Geneva
2. Butler MP et al (1999) Non-auditory effects of noise at work: a critical review of the literature post 1988. Sudbury, HSE Books
3. Bellieni et al (2003) Use of sound-absorbing panel to reduce noisy incubator reverberating effects. Biol Neonate 84:293–296
4. Probst R, Lonsbury-Martin BL, Martin GK (1991) A review of otoacoustic emissions. J Acoust Soc Am 89:2027–2067
5. Greenwood DD (1990) A cochlear frequency-position function for several species – 29 years later. J Acoust Soc Am 87:2592–2605
6. Moleti A, Sisto R (2003) Objective estimates of cochlear tuning by otoacoustic emission analysis. J Acoust Soc Am 113:423–429
7. Shera CA, Guinan JJ, Oxenham AJ (2002) Revised estimates of human cochlear tuning from otoacoustic and behavioral measurements. Proc Natl Acad Sci U S A 99:3318–3323
8. Abdala C (2000) Distortion product otoacoustic emission (2f1-f2) amplitude growth in human adults and neonates. J Acoust Soc Am 107:446–456
9. Kheifets L, Repacholi M, Saunders R, van Deventer E (2005) The sensitivity of children to electromagnetic fields. Pediatrics 116:e303–e313
10. Wertheimer N, Leeper E (1979) Electrical wiring configurations and childhood cancer. Am J Epidemiol 109:273–284
11. Bellieni CV, Rigato M, Fortunato M et al (2003) Increasing the engine–mattress distance in neonatal incubators: a way to decrease exposure of infants to electromagnetic fields. Ital J Pediatr 29:74–80

PART IV
Pain: a Risk Factor for Brain Damage

Chapter 14
Neonatal Stressors

M. Delivoria-Papadopoulos and O.P. Mishra

About 2.2 billion years ago, as the oxygen level of the planet was rising, a new sort of life form emerged, forged from a shaky alliance of what were to become the mitochondria and the remainder of the cell. The protomitochondria brought respiration to the partnership, and with it the power to kill every new cell by production of reactive oxygen species – a mechanism of cell death that still exists throughout the eukaryotes.

However, it was about 1.5 billion years later, as multicellular organisms emerged, that our story properly begins. Apoptosis has now evolved as a mechanism of physiological cell death in response to environmental and developmental signals. Apoptotic cell death is observed throughout the animal kingdom. Several recent advances have contributed to an emerging view of how apoptosis proceeds once initiated, to the point that we can speculate on a pathway for this remarkable process.

In the newborn, we are trying to find out the mechanisms by which the cell dies and brain damage occurs. But the most important part for clinicians is to understand the mechanisms of cell death not before hypoxia but after the hypoxia has occurred. Therefore, the aim of my discussion is to share with you experimental data to show how we have thought of asking and resolving some of the pertinent questions regarding posthypoxic brain damage and ways to learn to understand the mechanism.

Temporal Profile of Cerebral High-Energy Phosphates, Cell Membrane Na+-K+-ATPase, and Nuclear DNA Fragmentation Following Hypoxia

One of our main objectives was to evaluate biochemical changes over time and associated DNA fragmentation in the cerebral cortex of the newborn guinea pig following hypoxia. The experimental protocol was approved by the institutional Animal Care and Use Committee. We worked with pregnant guinea pigs so that we could control the timing of the birth of pups.

We divided the newborn guinea pigs into the following groups: the normoxic control, and the hypoxic group, where the guinea pigs were allowed to breathe 5–7% oxygen for 1 h. Following 1 h of hypoxia, the animals were studied either immediately or after 1 day, 3 days, or 7 days to answer the most crucial questions about delayed cell death in the brain. We measured the level of high-energy phosphates to assess the level of tissue hypoxia. We actually abandoned partial oxygen pressures because it is impossible to compare partial oxygen pressures when the hypoxic response of the animals is different in terms of adaptation. Accurate measurement of the levels of ATP and phosphocreatine in the tissues allows us to compare tissue hypoxia amongst several groups of animals and across several studies.

We started by measuring the cell membrane function of the neurons and Na^+-K^+-ATPase activity was one of the basic measurements we did. Our aim was to determine the development of DNA fragmentation. The following presentation examines first the results of our three groups of animals, particularly those at 7 days after hypoxia. After 1 h of hypoxia the ATP levels are significantly decreased, and 7 days later, although there is a tendency for ATP to come up, the level is still decreased and statistically different from corresponding normoxic controls.

Phosphocreatine responded in a similar way. There is a significant decrease in phosphocreatine immediately after 1 h of hypoxia that persists throughout the 7 days. At 7 days, despite a slight increase, it is still significantly lower than in normal controls.

Na^+-K^+-ATPase activity decreased during hypoxia and 7 days later was still decreased, although not statistically different for the number of animals studied.

The DNA fragmentation pattern was very clear. In the normoxic samples there is a presence of large fragments of DNA along with an absence of small DNA fragments. In the hypoxic samples, the low-molecular-weight fragments are present at 7 days, indicating that there was significant and dramatic fragmentation of the DNA 7 days after hypoxia.

This particular study can be summarized as follows: hypoxia resulted in a decrease in the cerebral level of high-energy phosphates, decreased cellular membrane Na^+-K^+-ATPase activity, and increased cerebral cortical nuclear DNA fragmentation, and 24–72 h following hypoxia the levels of high-energy phosphates and DNA fragmentation were slightly improved, but at 7 days the level of high-energy phosphates decreased, Na^+-K^+-ATPase activity was lower, and DNA fragmentation had increased significantly. We conclude from these studies that despite an apparent initial recovery following hypoxia, perturbations in cerebral energy metabolism, brain cell membrane function, and cerebral cortical nuclear DNA structure persist in the newborn guinea-pig brain. We speculate that a biphasic temporal pattern of the brain dysfunction following hypoxia may represent an initial cellular injury followed by a failure of cellular repair mechanisms, leading to further, delayed brain injury.

Temporal Profile of Neuronal Nuclear Ca^{2+} Influx and Expression of Proapoptotic and Antiapoptotic Proteins Following Hypoxia

A number of events occur inside the nucleus, including signal transductions that lead to apoptotic cell death. In the next several studies our objective was to evaluate changes over time in Ca^{2+} influx and Bax and Bcl-2 protein expression in neuronal nuclei of the newborn guinea pig following hypoxia.

Proteins of the Bcl-2 family are known to be critical regulators of programmed cell death and are expressed in neurons of the central and peripheral nervous system [1, 2]. The Bcl-2 protein, which is antiapoptotic in nature and was discovered in association with follicular lymphoma, regulates apoptosis and enhances cell survival in response to diverse apoptotic stimuli [3–6]. Bcl-2 family proteins have been shown by electron microscopy to reside in the nuclear envelope, parts of the endoplasmic reticulum, cytosol, and outer mitochondrial membranes [7–9]. Conversely, overexpression of the proapoptotic proteins such as Bax has been shown to promote cell death by activating caspases [10–12]. The active form of Bcl-2 heterodimerizes with Bax and their relative ratio appears to determine cellular susceptibility to apoptotic stimuli [12–15]. Bax and Bcl-2 are thought to play a role in cell death following hypoxia and ischemia. Studies have shown that cerebral hypoxia and ischemia alter the expression of these proteins [1, 3, 7, 14, 16, 17]. Studies have also suggested that Bcl-2 may suppress apoptosis by regulating cytosolic and intranuclear Ca^{2+} concentrations [18]. Nuclear Ca^{2+} signals control a number of critical nuclear functions, including transcription, DNA replication, and nuclear envelope breakdown [19–22].

The Ca^{2+} influx into the neuronal nuclei and the ATP-dependent Ca^{2+} influx will be the most important signal for molecular dysfunction. In addition, we focused on the apoptotic proteins, Bax and Bcl-2. The ATP and phosphocreatine decreased in the hypoxic group. However, we focused on the neuronal nuclear Ca^{2+} influx. We have shown before that during hypoxia Ca^{2+} influx into the nucleus increases and the mechanisms are in place that facilitate that influx within the nucleus. One day after hypoxia, there is a further increase in Ca^{2+} influx. Three days later it is still high, but 7 days later it is very impressive to note that the Ca^{2+} influx is at its maximum. The proapoptotic protein Bax increased after 24 h following hypoxia. At 72 h it was further increased, and 7 days later it was increased by 66% compared to controls. In contrast, Bcl-2, which is an antiapoptotic protein that maintains a cell life, did not change throughout normoxic states and hypoxic states longitudinally.

In summary, these studies showed that the neuronal nuclear Ca^{2+} influx increases in the postnatal period up to 7 days of age; that hypoxia results in an increased Ca^{2+} influx that remains elevated; and that the nuclear Bax protein expression increases immediately after hypoxia and remains elevated for 7 days while Bcl-2 protein expression remains unchanged.

We concluded that alterations in neuronal nuclear Ca^{2+} influx after hypoxia and Bax protein expression persist in the newborn guinea-pig brain. We speculate that alterations in the nuclear Ca^{2+} influx and the increased ratio of Bax to Bcl-2 proteins during the posthypoxic period promote delayed programmed neuronal death.

Effect of Allopurinol Administration on the Expression of Apoptotic Proteins and the Activation of Caspases

We can never deduce a concept unless we can eliminate, block, or intercept early steps. To achieve that, we utilized allopurinol, a xanthine-oxidase inhibitor. Studies have shown the therapeutic interventions of allopurinol, magnesium, and other substances that inhibit various steps of the apoptotic pathway. We used this inhibitor to prove our point, because if allopurinol inhibits the cascade of events, that would confirm the sequence of cell death mechanism that we have proposed.

We administered allopurinol to newborn guinea pigs to examine the effect of allopurinol administration after hypoxic changes in Bax and Bcl-2 and determined caspase-3 protein expression in the newborn.

Caspases are essential enzymes used for the normal development of the central nervous system. Caspases are cysteine proteases which contain a cysteine residue within their active site and cleave the peptide bond C-terminal to an aspartic acid of the substrate [23–26]. Like many other proteins, caspases are produced as procaspases (the inactive zymogen form) which are then converted to active enzymes following a proteolytic cleavage. Structurally, all procaspases contain a highly homologous protease domain, the signature motif of this family of proteases. The protease domain is divided into two subunits, a large subunit of approximately 20 kDa (p20) and a small subunit of approximately 10 kDa (p10). In addition, there is often a small linker region (about 10 amino acids long) between the two subunits. In addition to the large and small subunits, each procaspase contains a prodomain or NH_2-terminal peptide of variable length. It is this prodomain which contains the caspase recruitment domain (CARD). A charge–charge interaction controls the CARD–CARD interaction. Studies have shown that active caspases such as caspase-1 and caspase-3 contain the large and small subunits which are released from their respective procaspases through proteolytic cleavage, and both subunits are required for caspase activity [27, 28]. Studies have also shown that an active caspase is a tetramer (homodimer of the p20 and p10 heterodimers arranged in two-fold rotational symmetry), with the two adjacent small subunits surrounded by two large subunits [29]. These two heterodimers associate with each other through the interaction between the p10 subunits.

Caspase tetramers have two cavity-shaped active sites which function independently. In the active site, a cysteine (Cys-285 in the p20) is positioned close to the imidazole of histidine (His-237, p20), which attracts the proton from the cysteine and enhances its nucleophilic property. Caspase-9 is synthesized as a 46 kDa precursor protein. Like other caspases, it consists of three domains: an N-terminal prodomain, a large subunit (20 kDa/p20) and a small subunit (10 kDa/p10). Caspase-9 shares 31% sequence identity with the *Caenorhabditis elegans* cell death protein Ced-3 and 29% sequence identity with caspase-3. It contains an active site QACGG instead of QACRG pentapeptide which is conserved in other caspase members.

Caspases are a group of cysteine proteases that are essential for initiating and executing programmed cell death [30–35]. The activity of cysteine proteases is detected in cells undergoing programmed cell death, irrespective of their origin or the death stimuli. Studies conducted in *C. elegans* have demonstrated that an aspartate-specific cysteine protease is essential for programmed cell death of all somatic cells during development [36–38]. Mice lacking caspase-3 or caspase-9 have increased numbers of neurons in the brain and their lymphocytes are resistant to apoptotic stimuli [39–42]. Furthermore, the expression of baculovirus protein, a potent inhibitor of all known caspases, prevented developmental programmed cell death in *C. elegans* and in a number of cell lines [43–47]. Thus, it has been well established that caspases are critical regulators of cell death initiation as well as executioners of programmed cell death.

Once again in our experimental studies we used high-energy phosphates to assess hypoxia. We determined expression of Bax, Bcl-2, and the activity of caspase. We documented again the level of hypoxia by ATP and phosphocreatine and the activity of caspase-3, the executioner caspase. The activity of caspase-3 increased significantly during hypoxia and remained high during the posthypoxic period.

Bax is hardly visible in normoxia; it increases in hypoxia and 24 h after hypoxia as shown before. However, following administration of allopurinol after hypoxia, Bax is lower than the posthypoxic level, and definitely lower after 24 hours. Bcl-2 did not change. The active caspase-3 did not change after an increase following hypoxia and remained the same throughout. Bax increased during the 24 h posthypoxia and it is decreased in the allopurinol-treated hypoxic group.

To sum up, the findings of these studies were:
- That nuclear Bax protein expression increased immediately following hypoxia and remained elevated 24 h after hypoxia.
- That allopurinol attenuated the increase in the nuclear Bax protein expression that was observed immediately after hypoxia and at 24 h after hypoxia.
- That the Bcl-2 protein remained unchanged, and caspase-3 expression remained unchanged after it was increased after hypoxia.
- That allopurinol did not affect the increase in caspase-3 expression.

The speculation was that allopurinol pretreatment prevents alterations of the Bax to Bcl-2 protein ratio following hypoxia and may attenuate delayed neuronal death by a mechanism independent of caspase-3.

Effect of Allopurinol Administration on Neuronal Nuclear Ca²⁺/Calmodulin-Dependent Protein Kinase IV and Nuclear DNA Fragmentation

We examined neuronal nuclear protein kinase IV, which is a Ca^{2+}/calmodulin-dependent (CaM kinase IV) enzyme. This is a key enzyme in the transcription of apoptotic proteins. We determined whether pretreatment with allopurinol would attenuate posthypoxic alteration in the neuronal Ca^{2+} and CaM kinase IV activity. After hypoxia, the nuclear enzyme CaM kinase IV increased significantly. Twenty-four hours later it appeared low, but hypoxia plus allopurinol showed a significant difference.

Posthypoxic treatment with a low dose of allopurinol (20 mg/kg body weight) did not show an effect. Posthypoxic treatment with a high dose of allopurinol (100 mg/kg body weight) significantly decreased Bax without affecting Bcl-2. 24 h later there is a smear, 24 h of hypoxia and allopurinol show that there is still presence of fragments, but 72 h later there are fewer fragments of DNA even after post-allopurinol treatment. This was shown at the 7th day, when the fragments are much less and the last two panels, which are 7 days after hypoxia post-allopurinol treatment, look almost like the first two samples, which are normoxic. The DNA fragmentation shows very clearly; the squares are the hypoxic and with allopurinol treatment in which fragmentation decreases while in hypoxia it goes up.

In summary: in the cerebral cortex of newborn guinea pigs, nuclear Bax protein expression increases immediately after hypoxia and remains elevated at 24 h. A further increase is observed at 7 days. Allopurinol treatment following hypoxia prevented the increase in nuclear Bax protein expression observed at 7 days after hypoxia. Bcl-2 protein expression does not change. DNA fragmentation was observed following hypoxia and was decreased at 72 h, but increased fragmentation was again observed at 7 days after hypoxia. Allopurinol treatment following hypoxia attenuated the increase in DNA fragmentation observed at 7 days after hypoxia.

We speculate that treatment with allopurinol following hypoxia prevents alteration in the Bax to Bcl-2 ratio and may attenuate delayed posthypoxic neuronal apoptosis. The proposed sequence of events is this: with the influx of Ca^{2+} inside the cell, there is transformation within the intracellular space of xanthine-dehydrogenase to xanthine-oxidase, which is obliterated or inhibited by allopurinol. Thus, free radicals that otherwise would promote lipid peroxidation of nuclear membranes, enhance intranuclear Ca^{2+} flux and activate CaM kinase IV, which would phosphorylate the cyclic AMP response element binding protein molecule, which subsequently transcribes Bax and Bcl-2 genes.

In ending, I would like to point out that this is the tip of the iceberg and that a lot of work is still needed in order to see the exact sequence of the apoptotic pathway before we can dream and think of being able to inhibit it therapeutically. These inhibitions only prove the scientific value of the sequence of apoptotic pathways.

References

1. Chen J, Graham SH, Nakayama M et al (1997) Apoptosis repressor genes Bcl-2 and Bcl-x-long are expressed in the rat brain following global ischemia. J Cereb Blood Flow Metab 17:2–10
2. Merry DE, Veis EDJ, Hickey WF, Korsmeyer SJ (1994) Bcl-2 protein expression is widespread in the developing nervous system and retained in the adult PNS. Development 120:301–311
3. Chen J, Graham SH, Chan PH et al (1995) Bcl-2 is expressed in neurons that survive focal ischemia in rat. Neuroreport 6:394–398
4. Jacobson MD, Raff MC (1995) Programmed cell death and Bcl-2 protection in very low oxygen. Nature 374:814–816
5. Martinou JC, Dubois-Dauphin M, Staple JR et al (1994) Overexpression of Bcl-2 in transgenic mice protects neurons from naturally occurring cell death and experimental ischemia. Neuron 13:1017–1030
6. Zhong LT, Sarafian T, Kane DJ et al (1993) Bcl-2 inhibits death of central neural cells induced by multiple agents. Proc Natl Acad Sci 90:4533–4537
7. Hara A, Iwai T, Niwa M et al (1996) Immunohistochemical detection of Bax and Bcl-2 proteins in gerbil hippocampus following transient forebrain ischemia. Brain Res 711:249–253
8. Reed JC (1994) Bcl-2 and the regulation of programmed cell death. J Cell Biol 124:1–6
9. Rosenbaum DM, Michaelson M, Batter DK et al (1994) Evidence for hypoxia-induced, programmed cell death of culture neurons. Ann Neurol 36:864–870
10. Chinnaiyan AM, O'Rourke K, Lane BR, Dixit VM (1997) Interaction of CED-4 with CED-3 and CED-9: a molecular framework for cell death. Science 275:1122–1126
11. Golstein P (1997) Controlling cell death. Science 275:1081–1082
12. Krajewski S, Mal JK, Krajewska M et al (1995) Upregulation of Bax protein levels in neurons following cerebral ischemia. J Neurosci 15:6364–6376
13. Gillardon F, Wickert H, Zimmerman M (1995) Up-regulation of Bax and down-regulation of Bcl-2 is associated with kainite-induced apoptosis in mouse brain. Neurosci Lett 192:85–88
14. Gillardon F, Lenz C, Waschke KF et al (1996) Altered expression of Bcl-2, Bcl-X, Bax, and c-Fos colocalizes with DNA fragmentation and ischemic cell damage following middle cerebral artery occlusion in rats. Mol Brain Res 40:254–260
15. Oltvai ZN, Milliman CL, Korsmeyer SJ (1993) Bcl-2 heterodimerizes in vivo with a conserved homolog, Bax, that accelerates programmed cell death. Cell 74:609–619
16. Bossenmeyer C, Chihab R, Muller S et al (1997) Differential expression of specific proteins associated with apoptosis (Bax) or cell survival (Bcl-2, HSP70, HSP105) after short and long-term hypoxia in cultured central neurons. Pediatr Res 41:41A
17. Ravishankar S, Ashraf QM, Fritz K et al (2001) Expression of Bax and Bcl-2 proteins during hypoxia in cerebral cortical neuronal nuclei of newborn piglets: effect of administration of magnesium sulfate. Brain Res 901:23–29
18. Marin MC, Fernandez A, Bick RJ et al (1996) Apoptosis suppression by Bcl-2 is correlated with regulation of nuclear and cytosolic Ca^{2+}. Oncogene 12:2259–2266
19. Al-Mohanna FA, Caddy KWT, Boisover SR (1994) The nucleus is isolated from large cytosolic calcium ion changes. Nature 367:745–750
20. Santella L, Carafoli E (1997) Calcium signaling in cell nucleus. FASEB J 11:1091–1109
21. Steinhardt RA, Alderton J (1988) Intracellular free calcium rise triggers nuclear envelope breakdown in the sea urchin embryo. Nature 332:364–366
22. Tombes RM, Simerly C, Borisy GG, Schatten G (1992) Meiosis, egg activation, and nuclear envelope breakdown are differentially reliant on Ca^{2+}, whereas germinal vesicle breakdown is Ca^{2+} independent in the mouse oocyte. J Cell Biol 117:799–811
23. Mishra OP, Delivoria-Papadopoulos M (2002) Nitric oxide-mediated Ca^{++}-influx in neuronal nuclei and cortical synaptosomes of normoxic and hypoxic newborn piglets. Neurosci Lett 318:93–97

24. Alnemri ES, Livingston DJ, Nicholson DW et al (1996) Human ICE/CED-3 protease nomemclature. Cell 87:171
25. Donepudi M, Grutter MG (2002) Structure and zymogen activation of caspases. Biophys Chem 101–102:145–154
26. Salvesen GS (2002) Caspases: opening the boxes and interpreting the arrows. Cell Death Differ 9:3–5
27. Nicholson DW, Ali A, Thornberry NA et al (1995) Identification and inhibition of the ICE/CED-3 protease necessary for mammalian apoptosis. Nature 376:37–43
28. Thornberry NA, Bull HG, Calaycay JR et al (1992) A novel heterodimeric cysteine protease is required for interleukin-1 beta processing in monocytes. Nature 356:768–774
29. Rotonda J, Nicholson DW, Fazil KM et al (1996) The three-dimensional structure of apopain/CPP32, a key mediator of apoptosis. Nat Struct Biol 3:619–625
30. Thornberry NA, Lazebnik Y (1998) Caspases: enemies within. Science 281:1312–1316
31. Kumar S, Lavin MF (1996) The ICE family of cysteine proteases as effectors of cell death. Cell Death Differ 3:255–267
32. Nicholson DW, Thornberry NA (1997) Caspases: killer proteases. Trends Biochem Sci 22:299–306
33. Grutter MG (2000) Caspases: key players in programmed cell death. Curr Opin Struct Biol 10:649–655
34. Cohen GM (1997) Caspases: the executioners of apoptosis. Biochem J 326:1–16
35. Strasser A, O'Connor L, Dixit VM (2000) Apoptosis signaling. Annu Rev Biochem 69:217–245
36. Ellis RE, Yuan J, Horvitz HR (1991) Mechanisms and functions of cell death. Annu Rev Cell Biol 7:663–698
37. Xue D, Shaham S, Horvitz HR (1996) The Caenorhabditis elegans cell-death protein CED-3 is a cysteine protease with substrate specificities similar to those of the human CPP32 protease. Genes Dev 10:1073–1083
38. Yuan J, Shaham S, Ledoux S et al (1993) The C. elegans cell death gene ced-3 encodes a protein similar to mammalian interleukin-1 beta-converting enzyme. Cell 75:641–652
39. Kuida K, Zheng TS, Na S et al (1996) Decreased apoptosis in the brain and premature lethality in CPP32-deficient mice. Nature 384:368–372
40. Woo M, Hakem R, Soengas MS et al (1998) Essential contribution of caspase-3/CPP32 to apoptosis and its associated nuclear changes. Genes Dev 12:806–819
41. Hakem R, Hakem A, Duncan GS, (1998) Differential requirement for caspase-9 in apoptotic pathways in vivo. Cell 94:339–352
42. Kuida K, Haydar TF, Kuan C-Y et al (1998) Reduced apoptosis and cytochrome c-mediated caspase activation in mice lacking caspase-9. Cell 94:325–337
43. Bump NJ, Hackett M, Hugunin M et al (1995) Inhibition of ICE family proteases by baculovirus antiapoptotic protein. Science 269:1885–1888
44. Sugimoto A, Friesen PD, Rothman JH (1994) Baculovirus p35 prevents developmentally programmed cell death and rescues a ced-9 mutant in the nematode Caenorhabditis elegans. EMBO J 13:2023–2028
45. Hay BA, Wolff T, Rubin GM (1994) Expression of baculovirus P35 prevents cell death in Drosophila. Development 120:2121–2129
46. Beidler DR, Tewari M, Friesen PD et al (1995) The baculovirus p35 protein inhibits Fas- and tumor necrosis factor-induced apoptosis. J Biol Chem 270:16426–16528
47. Datta R, Kojima H, Banach D et al (1997) Activation of a CrmA-insensitive, p35-sensitive pathway in ionizing radiation-induced apoptosis. J Biol Chem 272:1965–196

Chapter 15
New Insights into Neonatal Hypersensitivity

C.J. Woodbury

Introduction

The skin, the largest sensory epithelium of the body, plays a pivotal role in the home-ostasis of organisms and is densely innervated by a wide variety of sensory neurons that have evolved to safeguard its integrity. Nowhere is this more important than in newborns, whose immune systems are not yet fully mature and for whom skin damage can therefore have serious immediate and long-term impacts on the viability of the organism as well as overall function of the skin sensory system. Attesting to this early vulnerability, newborn mammals of all species, including man, display a pronounced hypersensitivity to tactile stimuli over a protracted post-natal period (reviewed in [1]). Throughout this period of cutaneous hypersensitivity, protective withdrawal reflexes exhibit inordinately low activation thresholds and thus can be triggered by relatively innocuous stimuli. Rather than representing a para-doxical, maladaptive behavioural response, this hypersensitivity is undoubtedly highly adaptive in view of the pivotal importance yet extreme vulnerability of the integument and its associated protective/immune functions during early ontogeny.

The mechanisms underlying this early hypersensitivity are poorly understood. It has long been held that such hypersensitivity was triggered by activation of tactile afferents, due to the low activation thresholds of withdrawal reflexes and the wide-spread belief that the pain system was not yet functional due to delayed development of nociceptors [1]. Indeed, tactile afferents have been thought to invade noci-ceptive-specific regions of the central nervous system early on and commandeer nociceptive circuitry, in effect serving in the capacity of nociceptors during early post-natal timepoints while nociceptors were still immature. However, recent findings contradict this widespread belief, providing new insight into the identity of the sensory neurons that underlie neonatal hypersensitivity.

Skin Sensory Neuron Diversity

Skin sensory neurons, whose cell bodies lie in the trigeminal and dorsal root ganglia (DRGs), represent the skin's first line of defence against potentially harmful environmental insults. These primary afferents constitute an exceedingly diverse constellation of functional phenotypes, the majority of which are tuned to respond selectively to discrete intensities of mechanical, thermal, or chemical stimuli ranging from innocuous to noxious, and relay this information to central circuitry [2]. This functional diversity is paralleled by a similarly striking diversity in anatomical, physiological, and molecular phenotypic properties of skin sensory neurons. A major challenge in sensory biology is to understand the relationships between these properties, and how and when this diversity comes about during development.

From adult studies, while many diverse properties have been shown to be correlated to varying degrees with the discrete functional attributes of sensory neurons, the sheer complexity of these multifaceted interrelationships has strained the utility of broad generalizations. For example, the peripheral axons of cutaneous afferents range in size from large-diameter, thickly myelinated (Aβ) fibres to small, thinly myelinated (Aδ) and unmyelinated (C) fibres. Large fibres have historically been equated with low-threshold mechanoreceptors (LTMRs, or tactile afferents), whereas Aδ and C fibres have historically been equated with nociceptive afferents [2]. This classical account represents an oversimplification, however, as many nociceptors conduct in the Aβ range, while the most exquisitely sensitive tactile afferents often conduct in the Aδ and C ranges. As will become evident below, failure to recognize these important exceptions has helped promulgate a number of major misconceptions surrounding the development and plasticity of the pain system.

Another area where generalizations may be of limited usefulness is in studies of the biophysical properties of sensory neurons. Intracellular recordings have revealed a diversity of somal action potential shapes among sensory neurons, from broad (i.e. long-duration) spikes with a characteristic hump or inflection on the falling limb of the spike, to narrow (i.e. short-duration) spikes lacking this inflection. Historically, these quantitative and qualitative attributes of spike shape have been widely viewed as strong predictors of afferent functional identity, with narrow uninflected spikes associated with tactile afferents (LTMRs) and broad inflected spikes associated with nociceptive afferents [3]. Recent work from our laboratory that has examined nociceptor properties at normal physiological temperatures, however, has raised caution concerning attempts to infer afferent identity solely on the basis of biophysical properties [4].

A strong functional correlate is evident in the morphology and laminar termination patterns of sensory neurons where information is relayed by these afferents to central circuits in the spinal dorsal horn. While there are again exceptions, in general the central arborizations of different functional subclasses of skin sensory neurons are highly stereotypical and correlated with afferent modality [5]. In particular, nociceptive afferents have been found to terminate predominantly in superficial dorsal horn laminae I and II, whereas tactile afferents exhibit non-overlapping terminations that remain deep to nociceptive afferents in laminae III-V.

How and when these highly stereotypical laminar termination patterns of skin sensory neurons come about during development is unclear. Neuroanatomical tract-tracing studies, which depend upon bulk application of tracers to label large populations of unidentified sensory neurons, suggest that large-diameter afferents are the first to penetrate into the spinal grey matter of embryos, followed a few days later by small-diameter afferents [6]. It has also been suggested on the basis of such studies that these early-arriving, large-diameter afferents bypass their normal appropriate targets to invade superficial "pain-specific" or nocireceptive laminae during early life [7]. These fibres have been widely assumed to be LTMRs on the basis of axonal diameter and central morphology. This invasion and occupation of pain-specific regions by LTMRs has been thought to extend over a protracted period that in rodents encompasses the first 3 weeks of post-natal life [1, 7]. The adult bulk-labelling pattern is not seen until the 3rd week of life, when these exuberant central arbours retract from superficial pain-specific regions (but see [8]). This has led to a widespread perception that tactile afferents are extremely plastic entities, capable of invading and activating pain circuits directly at different times throughout ontogeny.

During pre- and post-natal development, this invasion of pain circuits by tactile afferents is therefore thought to underlie the hypersensitivity to tactile stimuli seen among neonates. Interestingly, the low activation thresholds of cutaneous withdrawal reflexes extend to about the 3rd week of life, mirroring the time course of these exuberant central projections from tactile afferents. This plasticity of tactile afferents is thought to continue throughout life, with exuberant growth into superficial pain centres again occurring in adults following nerve injury and/or peripheral inflammation [9, 10]. The activation of pain circuits by LTMRs is thought to underlie various chronic pain syndromes, most notably tactile hypersensitivity and touch-evoked pain (mechanical allodynia), that are common sequelae of nerve injury and inflammation.

Studies of Individual, Physiologically Identified Afferents

An important consideration is that all of these previous conclusions have been based upon morphological studies of unidentified afferents, i.e. the identity or identities of the sensory neurons upon which these hypotheses are based is unknown. To gain a better understanding of the anatomical and physiological development of skin sensory neurons in early neonatal life, we developed an ex-vivo somatosensory system preparation wherein the activity of individual sensory neurons could be recorded and functionally identified using natural stimulation of intact terminals in the skin prior to intracellular labelling of the same afferents for anatomical analyses of central termination patterns [11, 12]. In this novel preparation from mice, the spinal cord, DRGs, and cutaneous nerves are isolated in continuity with their innervation territories in the skin. The somata of individual skin sensory neurons are then impaled in the DRG with micropipettes containing Neurobiotin. Somal action potentials are recorded for analysis of biophysical properties. The latency of action potentials to electrical nerve stimulation provides information on conduction velocity and fibre size. A variety of natural stimuli (e.g. mechanical, thermal, and chemical) are applied to the neuron's terminals in the skin to characterize the neuron's peripheral response properties and overall functional identity. Following characterization, Neurobiotin is then introduced iontophoretically into the cell and allowed to diffuse throughout the cytoplasm. The tissue is then fixed, sectioned, and processed using standard ABC/DAB techniques, enabling visualization of the entire neuron, including cell body, arborizations in the spinal cord, and frequently peripheral endings in the skin. In addition to anatomical and physiological phenotype, the molecular phenotype of the cell can also be examined using fluorescence immunocytochemical techniques to determine whether physiological properties (e.g. heat sensitivity) are correlated with molecular expression patterns [13, 14]. This preparation therefore provides unprecedented power to address issues surrounding afferent identity and plasticity stemming from a variety of manipulations in neonates as well as adults.

Neonatal Tactile Afferents

In studies of newborn mice, the results obtained with this preparation have been strikingly consistent. Low-threshold mechanoreceptors (i.e. tactile afferents) exhibit adult-like central projection patterns in neonates as early as 1 day after birth (the earliest timepoint examined); that is, they do not invade superficial pain-specific laminae during early post-natal life [11]. This result was found for multiple distinct classes of LTMRs, ranging from those that will develop thickly ($A\beta$) to those that will develop thinly myelinated axons ($A\delta$), and those that exhibit distinctly different responses to mechanical stimuli (i.e. phasic or tonic). In all cases, the central arbours of tactile afferents remained deep to the superficial dorsal horn, separated from the outermost marginal layer (lamina I) by a distinct gap; this gap was found to be occupied by the central terminals of unmyelinated (C) nociceptive afferents. Along with adult-like laminar termination patterns, LTMRs in neonates exhibit adult-like physiological properties as well, including narrow, uninflected somal spikes as in adults, and remarkably adult-like response properties to a variety of natural skin stimuli. These findings of appropriate, adult central projections in neonatal animals therefore contradict the widespread belief that neonatal hypersensitivity is the result of inappropriate central terminations of LTMRs.

If LTMRs are physically incapable of activating superficial pain circuits directly, what populations of sensory neurons might be responsible for the hypersensitivity of protective nociceptive withdrawal responses in neonates? Another important point to note is that myelinated nociceptors have been ignored in all previous studies. These fibres bind the same cholera toxin labels that have been used previously to argue for a "transient invasion" of myelinated fibre inputs into superficial pain-specific regions of the dorsal horn, yet the contribution of myelinated nociceptors to bulk-labelling patterns has been overlooked in previous studies. Here again, the use of this semi-intact ex-vivo preparation to study the early post-natal development of individual myelinated nociceptors has provided a number of important insights into neonatal pain [15].

Neonatal Myelinated Nociceptors

With this detailed approach, we found two basic types of myelinated nociceptors in neonates as exemplified in Fig. 1. One class, with the most slowly conducting axons (i.e. future Aδ fibres), exhibited the classical central morphology associated with myelinated nociceptors, with terminations primarily restricted to the most superficial layer (marginal layer, or lamina I) of the dorsal horn. In addition to lamina I terminations, however, these afferents also projected into the substantia gelatinosa (lamina II; Fig. 1a), the region widely perceived to contain only unmyelinated C-nociceptor terminations. The other basic morphology (Fig. 1b) was seen among a different subclass of myelinated nociceptors with relatively fast conducting axons, a population that has been largely ignored to date. Many of these exhibited conduction velocities that were as fast as future Aβ LTMRs. In neonates, this population of future Aβ nociceptors gave rise to dorsally recurving arbours that were similar in many respects to the classical "flame-shaped" arbours described for LTMRs that innervate hair follicles. Similar to the latter, the central arbours from this population of nociceptors arborized throughout deeper dorsal horn laminae (III–V). However, in contrast to LTMRs, the distinctive arbours of these nociceptors did not stop abruptly at the ventral limit of the substantia gelatinosa, but instead continued uninterrupted into more superficial pain-specific regions, with extensive projections throughout superficial pain-specific laminae (I and II). Interestingly, this distinctive morphology has been found to persist throughout adult life in both in vitro [15] and in vivo studies (unpublished observations). Therefore, rather than a transient developmental phenotype, this population would be expected to contribute to cutaneous sensation throughout life.

As with other nociceptors, these afferents responded tonically throughout the duration of maintained stimuli, and their response became increasingly vigorous to higher forces in a manner capable of encoding the intensity of stimuli [15]. Interestingly, many of these afferents exhibited surprisingly low activation thresholds to mechanical stimuli, and tonic discharges were seen to innocuous stimuli. While these earlier studies were restricted to mechanical characterization, more recent studies of these afferents in neonates have found that many are also sensitive to noxious heat as exemplified in Fig. 1c. Indeed, these afferents responded to heat in a manner indistinguishable, in terms of threshold and evoked discharge, from heat responses seen across the same population in adults. Thus, similar to findings with tactile afferents, these studies reveal that myelinated nociceptors are also adult-like in all major respects in early life. Furthermore, in view of their relatively low mechanical activation thresholds and projections to superficial pain-specific laminae in the dorsal horn, this neglected and poorly understood population probably represents the afferent limb underlying hypersensitivity seen among neonates.

The existence of this novel central morphology in normal adults is particularly noteworthy. That these inputs to the substantia gelatinosa are not revealed with bulk-labelling techniques indicates that the latter are not sufficiently sensitive for these purposes. Nevertheless, these dorsally recurving flame-shaped myelinated nociceptor

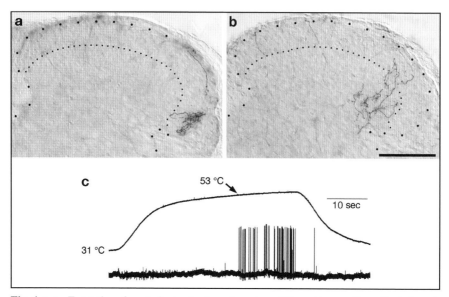

Fig. 1 a-c Examples of central arborizations from two different types of myelinated nociceptors innervating hairy skin in neonatal mice. **a** Slowly conducting (future Aδ) lamina-I/II-
specific myelinated nociceptor from a P2 neonate. **b** Fast-conducting (future Aβ) lamina I/V
myelinated nociceptor. *Large, widely spaced dotted lines* delineate the grey/white border of
the dorsal horn; *small, narrowly spaced dotted lines* delineate the ventral border of the substantia gelatinosa (i.e. lamina II). **c** Example of response to noxious heating of the receptive
field of a myelinated nociceptor from a P2 neonate. Note that the activation threshold was
53 °C, essentially identical to the average heat threshold (52 °C) for myelinated nociceptors
in adults. Responses to mechanical stimuli of this afferent are not shown; for examples, see
[11]. Scale bar (photomicrographs) = 100 μm

arbours are indistinguishable from those of the unidentified fibres interpreted as
"sprouted LTMRs" in earlier nerve injury studies [9, 10]. As with hypotheses that
invasion of tactile afferents into pain-specific regions of the dorsal horn could explain
hypersensitivity in newborns, the latter studies in adults suggested that the same
regions were invaded by these afferents again after injury, thereby explaining similar touch-evoked pain states. We now know this to be incorrect.

Inflammation in Newborns

While our recent findings from identified afferents have failed to support the major
tactile afferent plasticity invoked in these earlier scenarios, the possibility that such
plasticity may be present in nociceptive afferents remains a distinct possibility in
view of recent work involving damage and/or inflammation of the skin in newborns
[16]. We are currently examining this important issue in a mouse model of neonatal inflammation, and our results to date suggest that certain nociceptors are indeed

highly plastic and may be particularly vulnerable to early tissue damage as exemplified in Fig. 2. Inflammation at birth resulted in greatly expanded receptive fields among classical (i.e. lamina-I/II-specific) myelinated nociceptors; in some, innervation territories expanded to cover the entire innervation territory of the dorsal cutaneous nerve. By contrast, the receptive fields of these afferents in naïve animals are universally small and spot-like (Fig. 2a). Similar plasticity was also seen in the central terminals of these afferents as well, where arbours became highly disorganized and expanded into novel territories (Fig. 2b). Our findings so far have been restrict-

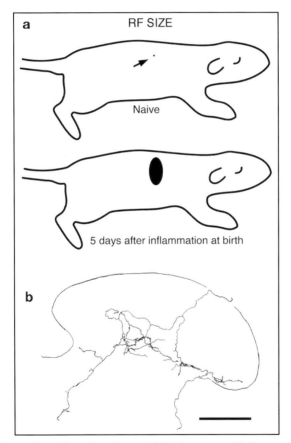

Fig. 2 a, b Changes in myelinated nociceptors following neonatal inflammation. **a** Schematic diagrams of neonatal mice (6 days after birth) showing approximate receptive field size of myelinated nociceptors in naïve, untreated animals (*small dot, top*) compared to animals that had experienced adjuvant-induced inflammation at birth (*large oval, bottom*). **b** Example of altered central projections from a myelinated nociceptor (5 days after birth) that had been exposed to adjuvant-induced inflammation at birth (compare to normal nociceptor arbours in Fig. 1); medial is to the *left*. Note the substantial disorganization and expansion of central arbours into somatotopically inappropriate regions of the dorsal horn; all normal afferents from dorsal cutaneous nerve nerves terminate in the lateral third of the dorsal horn. Scale bar = 100 μm

ed to the 1st week of life; whether these disruptive effects of neonatal tissue damage lead to permanent changes in the organization of the pain system is of considerable clinical importance and is currently being examined in long-term studies using this model.

Conclusions

These recent studies of the physiology and anatomy of identified skin sensory neurons have revealed that the skin sensory system is adult-like at birth. Tactile afferents in neonates are essentially miniaturized versions of their adult counterparts, and are not in a position to activate pain circuitry as previously believed. By contrast, myelinated nociceptors are also well developed early on, displaying thresholds to mechanical and noxious heat stimuli that are essentially indistinguishable from their adult counterparts. Unlike tactile afferents, however, these nociceptive afferents project extensively throughout superficial pain-specific laminae and can thus account for bulk-labelling patterns that were previously attributed to tactile afferents. The relatively low mechanical thresholds of certain subclasses of myelinated nociceptors can explain the marked hypersensitivity seen among neonates. However, as their mechanical thresholds are essentially identical to those seen in adults, the loss of neonatal hypersensitivity is likely to be due to alterations in central processing, and a potentially fruitful avenue for future research will be the examination of the development of central inhibition. Our recent studies also suggest that the nociceptive system may be particularly vulnerable to early inflammation and/or physical trauma. An important goal of future research will be to assess the long-term impact of this phenomenon and the molecular identity of the factors involved.

References

1. Fitzgerald M, Jennings E (1999) The postnatal development of spinal sensory processing. Proc Natl Acad Sci USA 96:7719–7722
2. Willis WD, Coggeshall RE (2004) Sensory mechanisms of the spinal cord. Plenum, New York
3. Koerber HR, Mendell LM (1992) Functional heterogeneity of dorsal root ganglion cells. In: Scott SA (ed) Sensory neurons. Oxford University Press, New York, pp 77–96
4. Boada MD, Woodbury CJ (2007) Physiological properties of mouse skin sensory neurons recorded intracellularly in vivo: temperature effects on somal membrane properties. J Neurophysiol 98:668-680
5. Fyffe REW (1992) Laminar organization of primary afferent terminations in the mammalian spinal cord. In: Scott SA (ed) Sensory neurons. Oxford University Press, New York, pp 131–139
6. Smith CL (1983) The development and postnatal organization of primary afferent projections to the rat thoracic spinal cord. J Comp Neurol 220:29–43
7. Fitzgerald M, Butcher T, Shortland P (1994) Developmental changes in the laminar ter-

mination of A fiber cutaneous sensory afferents in the rat spinal cord dorsal horn. J Comp Neurol 348:225–233

 8. Woodbury CJ, Ritter AM, Koerber HR (2000) On the problem of lamination in the superficial dorsal horn of mammals: a re-appraisal of the substantia gelatinosa in postnatal life. J Comp Neurol 417:88–102

 9. Woolf CJ, Shortland P, Coggeshall RE (1992) Peripheral nerve injury triggers central sprouting of myelinated afferents. Nature 355:71–77

10. Koerber HR, Mirnics K, Brown PB, Mendell LM (1994) Central sprouting and functional plasticity of regenerated primary afferents. J Neurosci 14:3655–3671

11. Woodbury CJ, Ritter AM, Koerber HR (2001) Central anatomy of individual rapidly adapting low-threshold mechanoreceptors innervating the "hairy" skin of newborn mice: early maturation of hair follicle afferents. J Comp Neurol 436:304–323

12. Koerber HR, Woodbury CJ (2002) Comprehensive phenotyping of skin sensory neurons using a novel ex vivo somatosensory system preparation. Physiol Behav 77:589–594

13. Woodbury CJ, Zwick M, Wang S et al (2004) Nociceptors lacking TRPV1 and TRPV2 have normal heat responses. J Neurosci 24:6410–6415

14. Albers KM, Woodbury CJ, Ritter AM et al (2006) Glial cell line-derived neurotrophic factor expression in skin alters the mechanical sensitivity of cutaneous nociceptors. J Neurosci 26:2981–2990

15. Woodbury CJ, Koerber HR (2003) Widespread projections from myelinated nociceptors throughout the substantia gelatinosa provide novel insights into neonatal hypersensitivity. J Neurosci 23:601–610

16. Ruda MA, Ling QD, Hohmann AG et al (2000) Altered nociceptive neuronal circuits after neonatal peripheral inflammation. Science 289:628–631

Chapter 16
From the Gate-Control Theory to Brain Programs for Neonatal Pain

K.J.S. Anand

Large numbers of low-birthweight (LBW) and preterm neonates are born in developed and underdeveloped countries each year [1], and many of them are extremely premature (<1500 g). For their normal, routine care it may be necessary for these infants to undergo repeated or prolonged exposure to stress, pain, and maternal separation in the Neonatal Intensive Care Unit (NICU). At this stage, the brain's architecture and vasculature are very immature, and these neonates can only survive because of improved obstetric and neonatal care [1]. Despite an increasing survival rate, preterm infants develop a high prevalence of cognitive deficits, learning difficulties, and abnormal behaviors during their early childhood and primary school years. Multiple follow-up studies of ex-preterm neonates have reported neurodevelopmental deficits [2–4], with needs for special assistance [5] and increasing burdens for health care and society [6].

We performed a meta-analysis on the cognitive and behavioral outcomes of ex-preterm children (cases) at school age compared to term-born children (controls), which showed that the mean IQ score of ex-preterm children is 11 points lower than that of children born from term pregnancies. The lower their gestational age and birthweight, the greater was the difference in mean IQ scores between the cases and controls [7]. Hack et al. showed a 5-point difference between the IQ scores of 8-year-old ex-preterm and term-born children, and this cognitive difference persisted until their follow-up at 20 years of age [8]. Despite their enormous significance for society, the biological mechanisms underlying these neurodevelopmental deficits remain unclear and underinvestigated.

Mechanisms Leading to Long-Term Effects of Pain and Stress

Neuronal cell death and altered synaptogenesis in the immature brain may offer plausible explanations for changes in cortical and subcortical brain regions noted from human and rodent studies. We investigated the mechanisms leading to these changes in order to explore the long-term effects of pain, stress, or other adverse experiences of the neonatal period. A theoretical framework [9] suggests that immature neurons and glial elements are vulnerable to apoptosis or excitotoxicity, and that repetitive pain or stress may have a significant impact on neuronal survival.

Enhanced Vulnerability of Immature Neurons

Brain development is critical just before and after human birth, which corresponds to the neurological maturity of 0- to 14-day-old rat pups, and is characterized by peak rates of brain growth [10], exuberant synaptogenesis [11], and expression of specific receptor populations. Neuronal receptors include the excitatory N-methyl-D-aspartate (NMDA) receptors, AMPA/kainate receptors, and metabotropic glutamate receptors, with widely distributed sites in the brain and key roles in neuronal proliferation, differentiation [12], migration [13], synaptogenesis [14], and synaptic plasticity in the immature brain [15]. NMDA receptors allow Ca^{2+} entry into the cell, which leads to phosphorylation of second messengers and changes in gene regulation. NMDA receptors reach a peak density at birth [16, 17] and are coupled with an increased magnitude of ligand-gated Ca^{2+} currents [18] in newborn rats. They are abundantly expressed in the human fetal brain as well [19]. Immature neurons appear to have greater vulnerability to excitotoxic damage [20], which may be due to altered molecular mechanisms for Ca^{2+} signaling [21]. This enhanced vulnerability of the immature nervous system, in the setting of increased stimulation by pathological stressors, may lead to an excessive amount of Ca^{2+} entry into the cell, which can initiate excitotoxic cell death. Prolonged blockade of NMDA receptors or the activation of neuronal cytokine receptors (e.g., the TNF-α receptor) may also trigger apoptosis in developing neurons [22], directly or indirectly, through the sequential activation of initiator (e.g., caspase-8, caspase-9) and effector caspases (e.g., caspase-3) [23–25]. This critical period is also characterized by enhanced degrees of naturally occurring neuronal death (or physiological cell death) via apoptotic mechanisms [26, 27]. Such neuronal cell death follows a developmental pattern, affecting particular brain regions during specific developmental phases, such as the brain stem in the perinatal period [28], thalamus and other subcortical areas soon after birth [29, 30], and cortical areas in the first 2 postnatal weeks [30–32]. The regional expression of Bcl-2 and caspase-3 appears to mediate this susceptibility to neuronal apoptosis, and this phase is terminated by the reduced cellular expression of caspase-3 [33]. In situ hybridization revealed a profound developmental regulation of caspase-3, the main effector enzyme for neuronal apoptosis, with a high abundance of caspase-3 mRNA observed in fetal and neonatal neurons and decreased expression in adult neurons [34]. Rabinowicz et al. calculated that large numbers of cortical neurons undergo apoptosis after 28 weeks of human gestation, with neuronal numbers decreasing by more than 50% to achieve a stable number of neurons at birth [26]. This vulnerability is not limited to neurons but extends to glial elements of the nervous system as well. Volpe and colleagues demonstrated that oligodendroglial cells present in premature human infants are exquisitely sensitive to free radical injury [35]. The predominant mechanism of oligodendroglial cell death occurs by apoptosis. This sensitivity to free radical injury is maturation-dependent, as mature oligodendroglia survive in much greater numbers when exposed to free radicals [36].

Effects of Early Adverse Experiences

The developmental regulation of excitotoxic and apoptotic mechanisms heightens the susceptibility of the immature nervous system to the adverse experiences in preterm neonates. Accordingly, models of hypoxic-ischemic injury in neonatal rats show increased neuronal necrosis in the cerebral cortex, striatum, thalamus, and hippocampus [37]. Viral infections of the neonatal mouse brain can cause increased cortical and hippocampal apoptosis [38], whereas remote stressors such as neonatal peritonitis also lead to neuronal and astrocytic injury, associated with impaired integrity of the blood-brain barrier in the frontal cortex [39]. Survival experiments further report a hyperresponsiveness of the hypothalamic-pituitary-adrenal (HPA) axis, correlated with permanent changes in the median eminence and hippocampus of adult rats following exposure to neonatal endotoxemia [40]. Neonatal intensive care aggressively treats hypoxia, hypoglycemia, or sepsis, but other factors contributing to neuronal damage, such as repetitive pain or maternal separation, have received little therapeutic attention until recently [41]. When the 8-year-old children studied by Peterson et al. were receiving neonatal intensive care, it was customary to ignore the effects of invasive procedures (e.g., heel lancing, venous catheterization, chest tube placement, etc.) or adverse environmental stimuli (e.g., loud noises, bright lights). Recent clinical and experimental observations suggest that the repetitive pain caused by invasive procedures, and maternal separation leading to a lack of social (tactile, kinesthetic, and verbal) stimulation, may have independent and perhaps inter-related [42] effects on the developmental vulnerability of immature neurons.

That repetitive or prolonged pain can insidiously hinder cognitive development has been largely ignored. For example, a similar pattern of long-term behavioral changes was noted in adult rats that were exposed to repetitive acute pain during the first postnatal week. Rats exposed to neonatal pain had lower pain thresholds during infancy, with increased alcohol preference, defensive withdrawal behavior, and hypervigilance noted during adulthood [43]. Neonatal rats subjected to inflammatory pain (induced by injection of formalin, complete Freund's adjuvant (CFA), or carrageenan) also manifested robust behavioral changes during adulthood. Following CFA injection in the neonatal period, adult rats were hyperresponsive to subsequent painful stimuli (pinch, formalin injection) [44]. Following exposure to repeated formalin injections, adult rats showed longer latencies to the hot plate, decreased alcohol preference, and diminished locomotor activity [45].

It is likely that these long-term behavioral changes may result from developmental alterations of the immature pain system at the peripheral, spinal, and supraspinal levels [41]. At the peripheral and spinal level these changes include increased sprouting of peripheral cutaneous nerves and their primary afferent connections with the dorsal horn of the spinal cord, corresponding to the area of tissue injury [44, 46]. Somatotopically related dorsal horn neurons showed a marked hyperexcitability, both at rest and following noxious stimulation, as well as decreases in their receptive field size [44, 47]. In the cortical areas associated with pain processing, it appears that repetitive inflammatory pain in neonatal rats leads to a significant accentuation of naturally occurring neuronal cell death [48]. Specific regions, particularly in areas of the piriform, temporal, and occipital cortex, show twice as many neurons dying in the 1-day-old and 7-day-old rats subjected to inflammatory pain as compared to age-matched controls, but this vulnerability was not evident in 14-day-old rat pups [48]. Mechanisms leading to these long-term changes may include neuronal excitotoxicity (mediated via activation of NMDA or other excitatory receptors) or apoptosis (mediated via inflammatory cytokine receptors or mitochondrial injury). NMDA-dependent mechanisms not only mediate the spinal transmission of pain but also the long-term effects of pain, such as hyperalgesia, allodynia, windup, and central sensitization [49], involved in the pathogenesis of chronic pain states [50, 51].

Accumulating data suggest that exposure to neonatal pain promotes an increased susceptibility to chronic pain states mediated by NMDA-dependent neuroplasticity [52, 53]. If neonatal pain or localized inflammation truly produce these long-term changes, then analgesia or anti-inflammatory treatment should prevent or ameliorate the expression of the reported cellular and behavioral changes. A paucity of published data, however, does not allow any firm conclusions in this regard. One recent experiment showed that pre-emptive analgesia with morphine in neonatal rats exposed to inflammatory pain reduced some, but not all the long-term behavioral changes noted in adult rats [45]. Preliminary evidence for the beneficial effects of pre-emptive morphine analgesia in preterm neonates comes from a blinded and placebo-controlled, randomized clinical trial, which suggests a reduced incidence of early neurological injury in the morphine-treated neonates [54]. The cognitive and neurobehavioral outcomes from a larger clinical trial (currently underway) may answer the question of whether the outcomes reported by Peterson et al. are altered by opioid analgesia, thus supporting the possibility that these changes resulted from pain-induced neuronal or white matter damage [55].

Summary and Conclusions

The neurodevelopmental outcomes of preterm neonates remain a cause for deep concern. We propose that NMDA-mediated excitotoxicity resulting from repetitive or prolonged pain and enhanced apoptosis due to maternal separation are the two primary mechanisms leading to enhanced neuronal cell death in the immature brain. Thus, neurodevelopmental abnormalities will depend on genetic variability as well as the timing, intensity, and duration of these adverse environmental experiences. Altered development during infancy may lead to reductions in hippocampal volume, abnormal behavioral and neuroendocrine regulation, and to poor cognitive outcomes during subsequent life. Ameliorating the subtle brain damage caused by these mechanisms may have a colossal public health and economic importance. Thus, concerted efforts by neuroscientists and clinicians to investigate the mechanisms underlying early neuronal stress, efforts to minimize the impact of adverse experiences in the neonatal period, and novel strategies for improving neurodevelopmental outcomes are justified.

References

1. Hoyert DL, Freedman MA, Strobino DM, Guyer B (2001) Annual summary of vital statistics: 2000. Pediatrics 108:1241–1255
2. McCormick MC, Gortmaker SL, Sobol AM (1990) Very low birth weight children: behavior problems and school difficulty in a national sample. J Pediatr 117:687–693
3. Breslau N, Chilcoat H, Del Dotto J et al (1996) Low birth weight and neurocognitive status at six years of age. Biol Psychiatr 40:389–397
4. Achenbach TM, Howell CT, Aoki MF, Rauh VA (1993) Nine-year outcome of the Vermont intervention program for low birth weight infants. Pediatrics 91:45–55
5. McCormick MC, Brooks-Gunn J, Workman-Daniels K et al (1992) The health and developmental status of very low-birth-weight children at school age. JAMA 267:2204–2208
6. Slonim AD, Patel KM, Ruttimann UE, Pollack MM (2000) The impact of prematurity: a perspective of pediatric intensive care units. Crit Care Med 28:848–853
7. Bhutta AT, Cleves MA, Casey PH et al (2002) Cognitive and behavioral outcomes of school-aged children who were born preterm: a meta-analysis. JAMA 288:728–737
8. Hack M, Flannery DJ, Schluchter M et al (2002) Outcomes in young adulthood for very-low-birthweight infants. N Engl J Med 346:149–157
9. Anand KJS (2000) Effects of perinatal pain. In: Mayer EA, Saper CB (eds) The biological basis for mind-body interactions. Elsevier Science, New York, pp 117–129
10. Rakic P (1998) Images in neuroscience. Brain development, VI: radial migration and cortical evolution. Am J Psychiatr 155:1150–1151
11. Rakic P, Bourgeois J-P, Eckenhoff MF et al (1986) Concurrent overproduction of synapses in diverse regions of the primate cerebral cortex. Science 232:232–235
12. Gould E, Cameron HA (1997) Early NMDA receptor blockade impairs defensive behavior and increases cell proliferation in the dentate gyrus of developing rats. Behav Neurosci 111:49–56
13. Komuro H, Rakic P (1998) Orchestration of neuronal migration by activity of ion channels, neurotransmitter receptors, and intracellular Ca^{2+} fluctuations. J Neurobiol 37:110–130
14. Yen L, Sibley JT, Constantine-Paton M (1995) Analysis of synaptic distribution within single retinal axonal arbors after chronic NMDA treatment. J Neurosci 15:4712–4725
15. Komuro H, Rakic P (1993) Modulation of neuronal migration by NMDA receptors. Science 260:95–97
16. Rao H, Jean A, Kessler JP (1997) Postnatal ontogeny of glutamate receptors in the rat nucleus tractus solitarii and ventrolateral medulla. J Auton Nerv Syst 65:25–32
17. Chahal H, D'Souza SW, Barson AJ, Slater P (1998) Modulation by magnesium of N-methyl-D-aspartate receptors in developing human brain. Arch Dis Child Fetal Neonatal Ed 78:F116–120
18. Mitani A, Watanabe M, Kataoka K (1998) Functional change of NMDA receptors related to enhancement of susceptibility to neurotoxicity in the developing pontine nucleus. J Neurosci 18:7941–7952
19. Ritter LM, Unis AS, Meador-Woodruff JH (2001) Ontogeny of ionotropic glutamate receptor expression in human fetal brain. Brain Res Dev Brain Res 127:123–133
20. McDonald JW, Silverstein FS, Johnston MV (1988) Neurotoxicity of N-methyl-D-aspartate is markedly enhanced in developing rat central nervous system. Brain Res 459:200–203

21. Ghosh A, Greenberg ME (1995) Calcium signaling in neurons: molecular mechanisms and cellular consequences. Science 268:239–247
22. Tsumoto T, Kimura F, Nishigori A (1990) A role of NMDA receptors and Ca2+ influx in synaptic plasticity in the developing visual cortex. Adv Exp Med Biol 268:173–180
23. Ikonomidou C, Bosch F, Miksa M et al (1999) Blockade of NMDA receptors and apoptotic neurodegeneration in the developing brain. Science 283:70–74
24. Du Y, Bales KR, Dodel RC et al (1997) Activation of a caspase 3-related cysteine protease is required for glutamate-mediated apoptosis of cultured cerebellar granule neurons. Proc Natl Acad Sci USA 94:11657–11662
25. Bonfoco E, Krainc D, Ankarcrona M et al (1995) Apoptosis and necrosis: two distinct events induced, respectively, by mild and intense insults with N-methyl-D-aspartate or nitric oxide/superoxide in cortical cell cultures. Proc Natl Acad Sci USA 92:7162–7166
26. Rabinowicz T, de Courten-Myers GM, Petetot JM et al (1996) Human cortex development: estimates of neuronal numbers indicate major loss late during gestation. J Neuropathol Exp Neurol 55:320–332
27. Dikranian K, Ishimaru MJ, Tenkova T et al (2001) Apoptosis in the in vivo mammalian forebrain. Neurobiol Dis 8:359–379
28. Miller MW, al-Ghoul WM (1993) Numbers of neurons in the developing principal sensory nucleus of the trigeminal nerve: enhanced survival of early-generated neurons over late-generated neurons. J Comp Neurol 330:491–501
29. Waite PM, Li L, Ashwell KW (1992) Developmental and lesion induced cell death in the rat ventrobasal complex. Neuroreport 3:485–488
30. Spreafico R, Frassoni C, Arcelli P et al (1995) In situ labeling of apoptotic cell death in the cerebral cortex and thalamus of rats during development. J Comp Neurol 363:281–295
31. Ferrer I, Bernet E, Soriano E et al (1990) Naturally occurring cell death in the cerebral cortex of the rat and removal of dead cells by transitory phagocytes. Neuroscience 39:451–458
32. Finlay BL, Slattery M (1983) Local differences in the amount of early cell death in neocortex predict adult local specializations. Science 219:1349–1351
33. Mooney S, Miller M (2000) Expression of bcl-2, bax, and caspase-3 in the brain of the developing rat. Dev Brain Res 123:103–117
34. Namura S, Zhu J, Fink K et al (1998) Activation and cleavage of caspase-3 in apoptosis induced by experimental cerebral ischemia. J Neurosci 18:3659–3668
35. Back SA, Gan X, Li Y et al (1998) Maturation dependent vulnerability of oligodendrocytes to oxidative stress-induced death caused by glutathione depletion. J Neurosci 18:6241–6253
36. Volpe JJ (2001) Neurobiology of periventricular leukomalacia in the premature infant. Pediatr Res 50:553–562
37. Nagata N, Saji M, Ito T et al (2000) Repetitive intermittent hypoxia-ischemia and brain damage in neonatal rats. Brain Dev 22:315–320
38. Despres P, Frenkiel MP, Ceccaldi PE et al (1998) Apoptosis in the mouse central nervous system in response to infection with mouse-neurovirulent dengue viruses. J Virol 72:823–829
39. Papadopoulos MC, Lamb FJ, Moss RF et al (1999) Faecal peritonitis causes oedema and neuronal injury in pig cerebral cortex. Clin Sci 96:461–466
40. Shanks N, Larocque S, Meaney MJ (1995) Neonatal endotoxin exposure alters the development of the hypothalamic-pituitary adrenal axis: early illness and later responsivity to stress. J Neurosci 15:376–384
41. Anand KJS (2000) Pain, plasticity, and premature birth: a prescription for permanent suffering? Nature Med 6:971–973
42. Gray L, Watt L, Blass EM (2000) Skin-to-skin contact is analgesic in healthy newborns. Pediatrics 105:e14
43. Anand KJS, Coskun V, Thrivikraman KV et al (1999) Long-term behavioral effects of repetitive pain in neonatal rat pups. Physiol Behav 66:627–637
44. Ruda MA, Ling Q-D, Hohmann AG et al (2000) Altered nociceptive neuronal circuits after neonatal peripheral inflammation. Science 289:628–631

45. Bhutta AT, Rovnaghi CR, Simpson PM et al (2001) Interactions of inflammatory pain and morphine treatment in infant rats: long-term behavioral effects. Physiol Behav 73:51–58
46. Reynolds ML, Fitzgerald M (1995) Long-term sensory hyperinnervation following neonatal skin wounds. J Comp Neurol 358:487–498
47. Rahman W, Fitzgerald M, Aynsley-Green A, Dickenson AH (1997) The effects of neonatal exposure to inflammation and/or morphine on neuronal responses and morphine analgesia in adult rats. In: Jensen TS, Turner JA, Wiesenfeld-Hallin Z (eds) Proceedings of the 8th World Congress on Pain. IASP Press, Seattle, pp 783–794
48. Newton BW, Rovnaghi CR, Narsinghani U et al (2000) Supraspinal fos expression may have neuroprotective effects in inflammation-induced neuronal cell death: a FluoroJade-B and C-fos study. Soc Neurosci Abstr 26(Pt 1):435
49. Kim YI, Na HS, Yoon YW et al (1997) NMDA receptors are important for both mechanical and thermal allodynia from peripheral nerve injury in rats. Neuroreport 8:2149–2153
50. Zhuo M (1998) NMDA receptor-dependent long term hyperalgesia after tail amputation in mice. Eur J Pharmacol 349:211–220
51. Baranauskas G, Nistri A (1998) Sensitization of pain pathways in the spinal cord: cellular mechanisms. Prog Neurobiol 54:349–365
52. Chiang CY, Hu JW, Sessle BJ (1997) NMDA receptor involvement in neuroplastic changes induced by neonatal capsaicin treatment in trigeminal nociceptive neurons. J Neurophysiol 78:2799–2803
53. McCormack K, Prather P, Chapleo C (1998) Some new insights into the effects of opioids in phasic and tonic nociceptive tests. Pain 78:79–98
54. Anand KJS, McIntosh N, Lagercrantz H et al (1999) Analgesia and sedation in ventilated preterm neonates: Results from the pilot N.O.P.A.I.N. trial. Arch Pediatr Adolesc Med 153:331–338
55. Peterson BS, Vohr B, Staib LH et al (2000) Regional brain volume abnormalities and long-term cognitive outcome in preterm infants. JAMA 284:1939–1947

PART V
Pain and Communication

Chapter 17
Disclosure of Pathology to the Newborn's Family

P. Arosio

Care of high-risk newborns often involves complex ethical problems, such as quick decisions about questions with a high degree of uncertainty. It is not always possible to define recovery, establish a long-term prognosis or predict future quality of life. This indicates the complexity of factors involved in relating to parents. I have been working for 20 years in the Neonatal and Intensive Care Unit of San Gerardo Hospital, Monza. I am also the president of an association of families with handicapped children (Gli Amici di Giovanni), which is affiliated with the national association "Famiglie per l'Accoglienza". I am not an expert in communicating, but all neonatologists have had to break "bad news", such as neonatal pathology, to parents, and have therefore had occasion to reflect on this experience. I shall touch on some points that seem important in the dynamics of communication between neonatologists and parents. I shall start with some data relating to my background experience.

Communicating a diagnosis means "making it *common*", entering into a relationship with the family and child. Communication of a diagnosis should not be an isolated event, but the first step in a therapeutic journey, a journey that should be planned and accompanied in the best possible manner for the parents.

Once the diagnosis has been communicated, the parents must not be left alone with their doubts, fears and anguish. They must be able to spend as much time as possible near their child and take part in the therapy. Open wards where parents can be present for most of the day are of great importance. However, the initial approach is crucial and can predispose parents to accepting or rejecting the baby (especially if affected by certain pathologies). For example, communication of an unexpected disease, such as Down syndrome to young parents, dashes the image of the awaited child. The doctor must try to have awareness and courage in being as little invasive as possible, creating affinity and empathy with the parents to enable the dialogue to continue.

To prepare this paper I used a letter that Dr. Bellieni wrote to me about 4 years ago, submitting a lesson of his to an up-dating course on neonatal care. The title of the lesson was "Who is the premature baby?". I remembered two points which are fundamental for entering into a relationship with the parents and for communicating the diagnosis [1]. It is not possible to talk of "what to do" or "what to say" to someone without having some idea of "who" that person is. Before being a clinical case or a set of symptoms, the newborn is a patient and a "you", a fragile you in a situation of great need and dependence [2]. This person or "you" cannot be conceived of outside a history, a family, a couple, without risking interrupting the continuity of a life made of sensations, smells, sounds, movements, that the baby is experiencing and experienced throughout fetal life [2]. We therefore have to think of the newborn within the unit it forms with its mother and father. I think it is helpful to bear these two points in mind when continuing the work of forming a relationship with the parents.

Let us now look at two aspects of the problem: the reaction of parents to communication of the diagnosis (Table 1) and the reaction of the doctor and how the doctor approaches this problem. The reactions of parents when told about the baby differ but follow a well-defined sequence of emotions which may vary in intensity and duration [3]. It is difficult to predict which reaction will prevail, and sometimes backward steps are made. The state of shock is a condition of confusion and impotence in which even the simplest information is difficult to grasp. It is followed by despair, sadness, disbelief (hope in a diagnostic error), anger and denial (when there may be confused hopes that the baby will die or hasty decisions to abandon the child). They are human reactions, understandable and even necessary, though not all are obligatory for the situation to mature and evolve towards acceptance and hopefully taking in (embracing) of the child. This phase becomes evident when the parents begin to see and describe their baby as it is (as it laughs or cries, sucks, sleeps or fusses) [4]. This experience eventually reinforces the couple. Reactions to the child may be characterised by conflicting emotions (over-protectiveness – coldness). Later, reactions towards the ward staff also develop [5].

Much also depends on the reactions of the doctor. Apart from their specific skills, doctors find themselves in a situation of stress, the intensity of which is related to the gravity, chronic nature or untreatable nature of the baby's condition and prognostic uncertainty. Our words and attitude should take account of the different prognostic implications of the pathology in question (Table 2). In

Table 1   Reaction of parents to news of an ill or malformed baby

Towards themselves	*Within the couple*
Shock	Trust
Blaming	Detachment
Despair	
Sadness	
Disbelief	
Anger	
Denial	
Taking responsibility	
Towards the baby	*Towards the staff*
Hyperprotection	Discharging tension
Medicalization	Absolute dependence
Alienation	Dissatisfaction

Table 2 Prognoses of some neonatal pathologies (modified from [3])

Good prognosis
Hypothyroidism
Adrenogenital syndrome
Congenital treatable cardiopathy
Uropathy due to malformation
Omphalocele

Uncertain, possibly good prognosis
Severe prematurity with possible sequelae (bronchopulmonary dysplasia, retinopathy of prematurity, brain haemorrhage with hydrocephalus)

Untreatable
Down syndrome
Severe intraparenchymal brain haemorrhage
Severe asphyxia

cases with good prognosis, the medical practitioner should explain the risks and benefits of therapy, reassuring the parents and eliciting their trust. When the prognosis is uncertain, possibly good, the doctor should sustain hope day by day, building trust in the treatment, in a therapeutic process that involves the parents and establishes human relationship. The figure of the doctor in charge of the case is important [6].

In cases where the pathology cannot be treated, it is more difficult to tell the parents and the emotional impact on them is greater. Much depends on the doctor's experience, including experience of life, and his or her attitude towards disease and handicap. Limitations may be encountered in this area. The parents are initially in a state of shock and confusion that makes them unable to fully grasp the information the doctor gives them; however, they will sense if the doctor is willing to understand and participate in their situation. Much of the work parents must do to receive and care for their child is mediated by us, our glances, our words and silences, an embracing or a cold and detached attitude. The way we look at the baby, the patient, is the same as the way we look at the people around us, our colleagues, the way we look at ourselves. Knowing this, some aims of communication (what to say, when and where to say it, and how to say it) can have a truer content, a less technical and certainly less sentimental form [7].

What to Say?

The truth is essential, but with how many details? In the case of pathologies with a rapid course, such as extreme prematurity with possible sequelae such as retinopathy and chronic lung disease, the truth should be told as it evolves, with doses and timing appropriate for parents undertaking a difficult and not always linear process, with its ups and downs, like the baby's pathology. The truth is our capacity to accompany the baby and its parents, observing timing that is not ours.

If possible, the diagnosis should be communicated to both parents, showing and giving them the baby. Reality is always less dramatic than imagination. Today the procedures of prenatal diagnosis have reduced the emotional trauma of communicating malformations or pathology at the moment of birth as many are diagnosed in utero and have already been communicated. Collaboration is necessary with obstetricians and gynaecologists so that the problem can be tackled together [8].

When and Where to Say It?

The diagnosis must be communicated as soon as possible and with every new development. It should be done in a suitable quiet place, to both parents and no one else, giving them the opportunity to freely express their feelings (including weeping) and to ask questions [9].

How to Say It?

This is the most difficult part and the one that most involves the doctor emotionally. Basically, it should be said with clarity and simplicity. Technical terms should be kept to a minimum, especially initially, on the first occasion. Parents more readily grasp the non-verbal dialogue, expressed through the attention and willingness of the doctor to understand and share what they are going through.

The facts should be presented as they stand, realistically. This seems a play on words, but is not intended as such. It should be done without prejudice and preconceptions that we doctors have sometimes borrowed from the media. It should be done with awareness of that unique "you" mentioned at the beginning.

Some optimism should be maintained, without denying the problems, but underlining the positive aspects and possible therapies.

References

1. Bellieni CV (1999) La Care in TIN: chi è il prematuro? Corso di Aggiornamento sulla Care neonatale. Siena
2. Brazy JE, Anderson BM, Becker PT, Becker M (2001) How parents of premature infants gather information and obtain support. Neonatal Netw 20:41–48
3. Burgio GR, Notarangelo LD (1999) La comunicazione in pediatria. Edizioni Utet
4. Coleman WL (1995) The first interview with a family. Pediatr Clin North Am 42:119–129

5. Cox C, Bialoskurski M (2001) Neonatal intensive care: communication and attachment. Br J Nurs 10:668–676
6. Fowlie PW, Delahunty C, Tarnow-Mordi WO (1998) What do doctors record in the medical notes following discussion with the parents of sick premature infants? Eur J Pediatr 157:63–65
7. Giussani L (1995) Alla ricerca del volto umano. Edizioni Rizzoli
8. Mastroiacovo PP et al (1986) Le malformazioni congenite. Medico e Bambino 5:
9. Jankovic M (1999) Come parlare ai bambini della loro malattia. Prospettive in Pediatria 29:61–66

Chapter 18
Communication of Diagnosis: Pain and Grief in the Experience of Parents of Children with a Congenital Malformation

L. Memo, E. Basile, A. Ferrarini, O.S. Saia and A. Selicorni

The majority of families who have children with a congenital malformation do not learn of their children's diagnosis until after the children are born, so breaking the difficult news of an unexpected diagnosis to parents in the newborn setting is a common occurrence for neonatologist. Presenting the diagnosis to families must be accomplished in a supportive, positive, caring, and honest manner. However, there are few scientific data and little instruction in training programs on how best to convey the news in an appropriate manner. Some articles in the literature over the last 30 years have proposed various guidelines for the so-called informing interview [1]. Discussions of parents' preferences and experiences in receiving this news have also been documented. Few reports, however, have focused on the breaking of the difficult news of diagnosis of a genetic condition to parents in the newborn setting [2–5].

Communication of a diagnosis is a particularly delicate and stressful moment: parents remember it for years. The communication process itself is extremely difficult; the parents are faced with a diagnosis of malformation and must cope with the manner in which they react, adapt, accept the child and modify their personal and family life. Many parents do not remember very accurately the specific contents of the communication or report that they did not understand. This difficulty, which is partially explained by the scientific nature of the information, underlines the importance of the emotional components of the interview.

Congenital syndromes are very complex and heterogeneous. It is difficult to define the possible reactions of parents. It is not possible to identify types of reaction in advance, because a syndrome or congenital anomaly is not the only variable which influences the parents' reactions. Some depend on the pathology, others on personality, on the quality of the parents' relationship, and on the sociocultural context in which the family lives. Appropriate management takes account of these different factors and the various phases of the process of adaptation [6–10].

The moment of birth and communication are a dramatic moment of shock which manifests itself in incredulity, disorientation, pain, a sense of impotence, and a blocking of the ability to reason. Pain and grief are always major feelings of the parents and always accompany the experiences of loss. Parents suffer from the loss of their "idealized child" and its assumed structural and genetic perfection. Sadness and anger follow pain and grief. In this situation it is important to support the family, helping the parents to process and overcome their sense of loss, with the aim of restoring family comfort and obtaining complete collaboration for diagnostic and therapeutic indications. After the first moments, a sense of negation and refusal are evident. These feelings cause defensive reactions and a sense of closure and failure. Overcoming of these first phases (coping) aids functional adaptation and a progressive ability to reorganize roles and the dynamic equilibrium of the family.

In this context, communication of a pathological condition is a fundamental moment. The experiences of some parents are complicated and deep:

"When she was born they told me that she was a beautiful child; I did not accept this, because it was not the truth."

"They give you the news and then they leave you alone, you don't know anything."

"They said very little, very quickly, about everything our baby was showing."

In a study in which 170 parents of children with a congenital syndrome answered a clinical–psychological questionnaire about how they received the information of their child's condition, the results showed that the news was extremely distressing and stressful in 53% of cases, hastily communicated and difficult to understand in 25%, and satisfactory as regards content and the manner of communication in only 15% (S. Intini, personal communication, National meeting of Italian CDLS Parent Support Group, Pesaro 2000).

At the moment when the news is broken, the effect of the emotions on the parents' rational ability prevents complete comprehension of the information. Unsatisfactory communication has a negative influence on the emotions and psychological feelings of the parents, and this has consequences for clinical and diagnostic plans by reducing parent compliance. This can cause a break in the medical relationship and increase the time taken for examination and specialist consultations.

Important factors for proper communication are appropriate communicative techniques and adequate context. The information must be given without delay, in the presence of the parents and the baby, in a comfortable, quiet, private location with enough time and no interruptions, sitting close to the parents, face-to-face, making eye contact [11, 12]. The clinical picture must be described to the couple in a simple language, with careful choice of words and avoiding euphemisms, technical diagnostic terminology or medical jargon, giving an objective opinion and not a list of problems. After the first discussion, it is very important to plan subsequent meetings to gradually explain the various diagnostic elements and their possible developments. The different medical specialists involved in communication and first assessments must be properly coordinated. In many cases, direct and indirect psychological and emotional support must be offered during and after hospitalization of the baby in the intensive care unit.

Direct support is of the psychological type; the psychologist has a prescriptive and organizing role more than an interpretative one. This intervention must be directed at a realistic shared understanding of the child's problems, help in discussions with the parents and integration of these problems into the family. Indirect support involves the organization of "environmental therapy", to improve contact between mother and child and the collaboration of the parents in the therapy, and to help the parents choose a doctor and nurse as reference persons in the department.

The period after hospitalization has particular characteristics and must be properly organized. It must be planned in agreement with the parents and the external paediatrician. A precise follow-up programme must be offered; help in dealing with social services and any other bureaucratic organizational problems, and with any obvious emotional or psychological distress is also necessary. It is also important to identify a professional figure that coordinates these activities; this role could be filled by the external paediatrician, the neonatologist or the paediatrician who first examined the child. If possible, this person should be a paediatrician who specializes in genetic problems and is experienced in general paediatrics and clinical genetics. The external paediatrician should support the family through diagnosis to guarantee the activation of integrated physical rehabilitation and psychological services, to define programmes of treatment and follow-up, to identify the right specialists for the child's various medical problems and to suggest formal and informal social resources for the support of the family. Parents need to be aware of the social services available in their area in terms of specialized services for mothers and children with disabilities. Organizing this for them will ease the stress of searching through different referrals, providing supervision and fulfilment of their needs.

We recommend the development and establishment of an infrastructure within each hospital system that makes routine the provision of up-to-date and accurate information and referral to parent support groups and other, experienced parents of children with congenital anomalies. It is important for the couple to exchange practical information, receive support and share experiences with other in a like situation. Hinkson et al. [13] feel that disorder-specific support groups are crucial, since they are composed primarily of caregivers who have first-hand experience of caring for similarly affected children and can provide appropriate information that is most likely to match the changing concerns of others caregivers. The neonatologist and/or the paediatrician should provide the family with information about these types of association, leaving the parents free to decide themselves how and when to make contact.

References

1. Dent KM, Carey JC (2006) Breaking difficult news in a newborn setting: Down syndrome as a paradigm. Am J Med Genet C Semin Med Genet 142:173–179
2. Fallowfield L, Jenkins V (2004) Communicating sad, bad, and difficult news in medicine. Lancet 363:312–319
3. Krahn GL, Hallum A, Kime C (1993) Are there good ways to give "bad news"? Pediatrics 91:578–582
4. Ptacek JT, Eberhardt TL (1996) Breaking bad news. A review of literature. JAMA 276:496–502
5. Ryan S (1995) Telling parents their child has severe congenital anomalies. Postgrad Med J 71:529–533
6. Cunningham CC, Morgan PA, McGucken RB (1984) Down's syndrome: is dissatisfaction with disclosure of diagnosis inevitable? Dev Med Child Neurol 26:33–39

7. Cuskelly M, Gunn P (2003) Sibling relationships of children with Down syndrome: perspectives of mothers, fathers and siblings. Am J Ment Retard 108:234–244
8. Drotar D, Baskiewicz A, Irvin N et al (1975) The adaptation of parents to the birth of an infant with a congenital malformation: a hypothetical model. Pediatrics 56:710–717
9. Garwick AW, Patterson J, Bennet CF et al (1995) Breaking the news. How families first learn about their child's chronic condition. Arch Pediatr Adolesc Med 149:991–997
10. Hedov G, Wikblad K, Anneren G (2002) First information and support provided to parents of children with Down syndrome in Sweden: clinical goals and parental experiences. Acta Paediatr 91:1344–1349
11. Mastroiacovo PP, Memo L (2007) Raccomandazioni per la comunicazione della diagnosi di malattia genetica complessa e/o di disabilità congenita. Prospettive in Pediatria (in press)
12. Rosenthal ET, Biesecker LG, Biesecker BB (2001) Parental attitudes toward a diagnosis in children with unidentified multiple congenital anomaly syndromes. Am J Med Genet 103:106–114
13. Hinkson DAR, Atenafu E, Kennedy SJ et al (2006) Cornelia De Lange syndrome: parental preferences regarding the provision of medical information. Am J Med Genet 140A:2170–2179

Chapter 19
Invest in Prenatal Life: a High-Yield Stock

M. Enrichi

In the last 20 years various associations have been formed, inside and outside academic and health circles, to provide information on prenatal life and the importance of this special period for our physical and emotional life and relationships. Founded in 1992, ANEP (Associazione Nazionale Educazione Prenatale) is the Italian chapter of the Organisation Mondiale des Associations pour l'Education Prénatale (OMAEP), founded in France in 1982, which now contains 18 national associations. Another association, ANPEP (Associazione Nazionale Psicologia Educazione Prenatale), was founded in 1999. An understanding of prenatal life needs to become part of the cultural heritage, especially for couples planning to have a family or expecting a baby, and for school children. Thus the fascination of the first 9 months of life will leave a mark in the DNA of the heart, as well as in the personal cultural heritage that school inculcates in us all, and respect for life and its wonders will have a stronger foundation. Knowledge and respect for life, especially the bud of life, when it is so small as to seem insignificant and so defenceless as to seem in our power, can enable us to know our origins, which are the same for all of us – the basic equality – and need to be embraced in common by all of us, reinforcing ancient words of peace. Knowledge of prenatal life is therefore precious.

Prenatal life is a high-yield stock, because an increase in fetal health becomes an increase in adult health and because health is a basic right and social aim, especially at the start of life [1]. Investment in prenatal life pays because 9 months are worth a life. Prenatal life is a fundamental time for life because it is at the beginning. The environment, especially the mother's body, moulds prenatal development through experience. Experience is nourishment: biochemical, metabolic, sensory, cellular, emotional, relational, and cognitive.

The studies of Barker have shown that physiology and metabolism change permanently when the fetus has to adapt to an unfavourable environment, and that these programmed changes may underlie illness in adulthood [2]. The role of the environment is becoming increasingly recognized. It is increasingly evident that almost all illnesses have an environmental component, that the effect is much more harmful in the aetio-pathogenesis of disease if exposure to insult occurs during development, and that the outcome may be not only malformation but also functional deficit which may manifest later in life [3].

G. Buonocore, C.V. Bellieni (eds), *Neonatal Pain. Suffering, Pain and Risk of Brain Damage in the Fetus and Newborn*, © Springer 2008

Prenatal experience is also sensory experience. The work of Mauro Mancia, pioneer in the encounter between neuroscience and psychoanalysis, has shown that "sensoriality" – i.e. fetal sensory experience through integration of pons structures – underlies active sleep, stimulates synaptogenesis, determines implicit memory, participates in control of the vegetative system, and takes part in sensory transmodality. Active sleep is the nucleus of the baby's representational mode at birth; synaptogenesis is the process behind learning, memory, and intelligence, and hence the cognitive self. Implicit memory is the nucleus of the emotional self and the axis of the self, namely the emotional centre of personality. Sensory experience takes part in the control of the vegetative system, including heart and respiratory control, and is linked with postnatal life, as we shall see. Sensory experience is involved in sensory transmodality, which is the fetal and neonatal capacity to pass information from one channel to another [4]. Finally, emotional and sensory experience is the experience of suffering and pain, lived through the troubles and stress of the mother or directly in the fetal body, and its mark remains long after birth as many neuroendocrinological, neuropsychiatric, and neonatological studies show [5–7].

Studies in psychology and psychoanalysis show that maternal representations in pregnancy – that is, the idea the woman has of herself during pregnancy, as a pregnant woman and as a mother, that she has of the baby and the relationship between them (which underlie motherhood and bonding of the newborn and baby with its parent figures) – are the operative model through which adults form relationships [8–11]. These representations form a thread of continuity between pregnancy and the postnatal period. They are present from the start of pregnancy and are quite well formed in the second trimester, a crucial time in which their construction undergoes acceleration [9–11]. These representations can be revised during pregnancy as new information is acquired, and can therefore be modified [10].

Sensory experience is therefore a stimulus for sensorineuromotor construction. Sensory stimuli take part in the control of vegetative life before and after birth. It has been demonstrated that auditory input is important for maintaining diencephalic respiratory centre function. Auditory input in particular has a major role in regulation of breathing during neonatal sleep, to the extent that development of environmental acoustic stimuli is a major protective factor against cot death, as acoustic stimulation reduced the risk of central apnoea [12].

The fact that fetal cells pass into the maternal circulation during pregnancy has been known for over a century [13]. Recent studies indicate that cells transfer between fetus and mother during pregnancy and can persist in both decades later, almost life long [14]. The presence within one individual of a small population of cells from another genetically distinct individual is referred to as microchimerism [15]. A term pregnancy is not required for the development of fetal cell microchimerism, and for a woman to become a chimera following pregnancy [14].

Natural microchimerism is maternal (mother's cells in the fetus) and fetal (fetal cells in the mother) [14]. The potential role of such placental transfer is still unknown, but the finding of a high frequency of fetal microchimerism in the maternal liver suggests the possibility that this migration may be important in the induction and subsequent maintenance of tolerance towards the fetus during pregnancy [16]. Persisting maternal and fetal microchimerism could be involved in the induction of some autoimmune diseases [15]. Alternatively, maternal and fetal cells may migrate to areas of tissue damage secondarily and function beneficially in repair [13, 17]. The medical consequences of pregnancy, therefore, appear to extend well beyond delivery [18].

Psychiatrists and psychologists have long since brought to light the importance of the mother–child relationship in utero. Prenatal life sculpts one's personality on the basis of this relationship. The basic principle of the human being is to-be-in-relation, to-be-with, mit-sein, dialogue [19]. Every stimulus is relative. The stimulus and the reaction will become a component of the personality that is to be, becomes "biologic", a true imprinting that is there to stay and yields the "personality's sculpture". Every stimulus reaches the fetus and the fetus unfailingly reacts against the events reaching him; if they repeatedly trouble him they produce a "silent trauma", forcing the fetus to raise defensive barriers that require a continuous waste of energy [19]. The mother and the environment send messages that influence the fetus, his relation with his mother and the world around him, and his brain development [6]. Today stress is a subtle and ever-present toxin that when acting on a pregnant woman can cause premature birth and infantile psychopathologies [5]. Clinical studies in the third trimester of pregnancy have proved that an important stress is associated with a statistically significant risk of neurobehavioural dysfunctions [6]; that the first modality of "to-be-with" is built with the parents' emotional mood pattern [19]; that there is reciprocity between bonding (the parent's attachment toward the child) and attachment (the child's tendency to attachment) [20]; and there is a correlation between prenatal bonding and postnatal attachment [21].

Prenatal education is to let both parents know how important it is that they are parents, because:

- The father is always present, even when he is not, because he is in the mother's mind [22].
- The primary triangle (first relation mother–father–child) is present starting from the prenatal period [20].
- Triadic interactions (mother–father–child) arise early if the parents respond appropriately and if they create an ever-growing state of awareness; and if it is possible for there to be continuity in the interactive and affective organization between the prenatal and the postnatal period [20].

At this point we can draw some conclusions about the principles of prenatal education. First and foremost is the principle that every child is a miracle, and since these days we all talk by slogans, we will conclude with some slogans:

- For the mother: "Take care of yourself."
- For the father, family, and society: take care of the mother, prepare to welcome the baby. In other words: "Number one: ecology."
- For everyone: get to know prenatal life: "To know it is to love it."
- For the mother and the father: trust in your abilities and competence, and at the same time trust in the vital strength of the child: "Equal dignity."

- For the mother and the father: maximize all sensorial communications as much and as soon as possible: "It's never too early, it's never too late."

What can we do to invest in prenatal life? Apart from health policy and medical aspects, it is important that people be informed about prenatal life. Knowledge of prenatal life arouses a sense of wonder and rapture, potentiating the perception of fetal life as something precious and increasing respect for the developing embryo and the woman bearing it. This has many good repercussions, making pregnant women prefer a healthier and more appropriate life style. Couples also weave a richer and more complex relationship by thinking and caring about the baby. Finally, all of us and society itself begin to wish to create a more protective environment for the unborn baby and its mother.

We believe that all this can contribute to change the experience of prenatal life on which the life of adult humans is built.

References

1. International Conference on Primary Health Care (1978) Alma Ata, USSR, 6-12 September
2. Barker DJ (1995) The Wellcome Foundation Lecture, 1994. The fetal origins of adult disease. Proc R Soc Lond B Biol Sci 262(1363):37–43
3. The Fetal basis of adult disease: role of the environment Program Announcement (PA) (2002) National Institutes of Health, Bethesda, Maryland
4. Mancia M (2001) Organizzazione della mente infantile. Ruolo della vita prenatale e neonatale. In: Impatto della vita parentale sull'evoluzione dell'individuo, della cultura e della società. Proceedings of the Convegno Nazionale Associazione Nazionale Educazione Prenatale, Milan 9-10 June 2001, pp 9–11
5. Panzarino P (2003) Ruolo dello stress materno e delle altre influenze ambientali sullo sviluppo mentale del feto. In: Astrei G, Bevere A (eds) Vita prenatale e sviluppo della personalità. Cantagalli, Siena, pp 15–19
6. Ottaviano S, Ottaviano P, Ottaviano C (2003) Stress materno-fetale nel terzo trimestre di gravidanza, sindromi neurocomportamentali neonatali e PEP (Programmi Educativi Prenatali). In: Astrei G, Bevere A (eds) Vita prenatale e sviluppo della personalità. Cantagalli, Siena, pp 225–236
7. Bellieni CV (2002) Il dolore del Feto. In: Enrichi M (ed) 9 Mesi e un giorno. Proceedings of Congresso Scientifico Internazionale Università degli Studi La Sapienza e Associazione Nazionale Educazione Prenatale. Roma 18-19 Ottobre 2002, pp 11-15
8. Stern DN (1987) Il mondo interpersonale del bambino. Bollati-Boringhieri, Turin
9. Ammaniti M (1995) Le categorie delle rappresentazioni in gravidanza. In: Ammaniti M, Candelori C, Pola M, Tambelli R: Maternità e gravidanza. Studio delle rappresentazioni materne. Raffaello Cortina, Milan, pp 33–42
10. Tambelli R (1995) Una indagine sulle rappresentazioni in gravidanza. In: Ammaniti M, Candelori C, Pola M, Tambelli R: Maternità e gravidanza. Studio delle rappresentazioni materne. Raffaello Cortina, Milan, pp 43–62
11. Fava Vizziello G, Antonioli ME, Cocci V, Invernizzi R (1995) Dal mito al bambino reale. In: Ammaniti M (ed) La gravidanza tra fantasia e realtà. Pensiero scientifico, Rome, pp 159–180
12. Cosmi EV (2002) Trattamento del neonato pretermine con il metodo Kangaroo. Proceedings of Ninth National Congress of the Società Italiana di Medicina Perinatale (SIMP). Monduzzi, Bologna, pp 165–168

13. Schmorl G (1893) Pathologisch-anatomische Untersuchungen über Puerperal Eklampsie. Verlag von FC Vogel, Leipzig
14. Bianchi DW (2000) Feto-maternal cell trafficking: a new cause of disease? Am J Med Genet 91:22–28
15. Adams KM, Nelson JL (2004) Microchimerism: an investigative frontier in autoimmunity and transplantation. JAMA 291:1127–1131
16. Tanaka A, Lindor K, Ansari A, Gershwin ME (2000) Fetal microchimerism in the mother: immunological implications. Liver Transpl 6:138–143
17. Bianchi DW (2000) Fetal cells in the mother: from genetic diagnosis to disease associated with fetal cell micromerism. Eur J Obstet Gynecol Reprod Biol 92:103–108
18. Khosrotehrani K, Bianchi DW (2003) Fetal cells micromerism: helpful or harmful to the parous woman? Curr Opin Obstet Gynecol 15:195–199
19. Ancona L (2003) Impianto e sviluppo della personalità. In: Astrei G, Bevere A (eds) Vita prenatale e sviluppo della personalità. Cantagalli, Siena, p 21
20. Zavattini GC (2002) Psicodinamica degli affetti nella coppia: coniugalità e genitorialità. In: Enrichi M (ed) 9 Mesi e un giorno. Proceedings of Congresso Scientifico Internazionale Università degli Studi La Sapienza e Associazione Nazionale Educazione Prenatale. Roma 18-19 Ottobre 2002, p 101-111
21. Tambelli R, Odorisio F (2002) Le rappresentazioni materne e paterne in gravidanza e le relazioni precoci con il bambino. In: Enrichi M (ed) 9 Mesi e un giorno. Proceedings of Congresso Scientifico Internazionale Università degli Studi La Sapienza e Associazione Nazionale Educazione Prenatale. Roma 18-19 Ottobre 2002, p 121-125
22. Ammaniti M, Vismara L (2002) Dinamiche psichiche in gravidanza e sviluppo infantile precoce. In: Enrichi M (ed) 9 Mesi e un giorno. Proceedings of Congresso Scientifico Internazionale Università degli Studi La Sapienza e Associazione Nazionale Educazione Prenatale. Roma 18-19 Ottobre 2002, p 81-87

Subject Index